Praise for
Dissociation Made

T0049180

"Challenging many practices even within trauma-informed care, this book gives us the fresh approach we've needed to look at dissociation—and thus at addiction—in a way that challenges the status quo of treatment and the stigma around mental health and addiction."

—ANNA DAVID, *New York Times* best-selling author of *Party Girl* and founder of Legacy Launch Pad Publishing

"Jamie Marich brings her lived experiences forward in this bold new book. Both scientifically grounded and authentic in its expression, *Dissociation Made Simple* is a refreshing and necessary addition to the clinical discussion of trauma and dissociation."

—EMMA SUNSHAW, creator of the *System Speak* podcast and author of *If Tears Were Prayers*

"Dr. Jamie Marich is a pioneer in the trauma-recovery field. Her expert strategies are always accompanied by compassion and kindness. Her depth of knowledge means that you are always in good hands. I will recommend this book to my clients."

—VERONICA VALLI, author of *Soberful* and cohost of the *Soberful* podcast

"Jamie Marich's honesty about her personal experiences combined with her professional knowledge serve to demystify and de-pathologize a common adaptive survival response and to provide readers with hope and embodied self-compassion. *Dissociation Made Simple* balances neuroscience with a much-needed spiritual-injury lens often missing in clinical settings."

—JANE CLAPP, author and founder of Jungian Somatics

"*Dissociation Made Simple* takes an honest look at the realities dissociative survivors face—within and outside of the mental health care system. A helpful guide for both survivors and practitioners, this book normalizes dissociation as the brilliant, adaptive coping mechanism that it truly is. Thank you, Jamie, for your courage and commitment."

—ADRIAN A. FLETCHER, PsyD, MA, psychologist, writer, and empowerment speaker living and thriving with dissociative identities

"As a survivor of childhood sexual abuse and complex trauma with dissociative identity disorder (DID), I've been waiting for this book. Not only does it provide everyday tools and exercises, but it also allows you to feel and heal on a profound level. It is an indispensable resource. *Dissociation Made Simple* is a must-read across the broad spectrum of trauma-recovery work."

—LARRY RUHL, artist, advocate, and author of the best-selling memoir *Breaking the Ruhls*

"Dr. Jamie Marich is the rebel pilot that the trauma field desperately needs. Skillfully balancing research with personal narratives, *Dissociation Made Simple* is as informative as it is engaging. Dr. Marich invites readers to recognize the multiplicity of their own mind and to recognize that all humans dissociate and contain an inner multiverse. Whether this information is new or a familiar personal experience, all readers will find value in this book. The message is clear in the writing: all readers are welcome."

—JUSTINE MASTIN, MA, LMFT, LADC, E-RYT 200, coauthor of *Starship Therapise*

"*Dissociation Made Simple* pushes the mental health field to examine its definitions and labels, push past its limited psychotherapy-treatment options, and welcome expanded cross-cultural understanding and treatment approaches for people overcoming trauma. Marich provides a bridge between differing views with her unique ability to validate and honor what is working with current approaches while opening our eyes to new healing options for managing our complex human parts in response to daily life. Current Western treatment approaches and labels of 'disorder' have often left me and my clients feeling disempowered, defective, and disordered. This book offers solutions that empower, motivate, and inspire us to stay the course on our healing journey."

—ANNA PIRKL, coauthor of *Transforming Trauma with Jiu-Jitsu*

"If you are looking for a sensitive and respectful work on dissociation—one that shows that this challenging, complex subject is qualitatively researchable, one that enables the voices from the inside and the voices from the outside to be heard, to express themselves—you will find it here. This is the book for us."

—DR. ANDRÉ MAURÍCIO MONTEIRO, Espaço da mente, Brazil

"In this groundbreaking book, Dr. Jamie Marich brilliantly explains and simplifies a common phenomenon that so many people experience and struggle to understand. A must-read for anyone looking to improve their mental health and break free from the stigma of dissociation."

—ERICA HORNTHAL, LCPC, BC-DMT, author of *Body Aware*

"*Dissociation Made Simple* offers a comprehensive guide to understanding dissociation. Its emphasis on unpacking and demystifying this oft-misunderstood byproduct of trauma is particularly salient during a pandemic—when many have been retraumatized and more deeply entrenched in their *zoned-out* trauma-selves. Individuals and clinicians alike will find this guide useful. It approaches the topic on a human level with real-life examples, avoiding academic jargon and providing straightforward ways of looking at dissociation. Not only does Dr. Marich's book destigmatize dissociation, but it also offers a silver lining to those who live with it—the gifts of dissociation."

—ANN GOELITZ, PhD, LCSW, author of *From Trauma to Healing*

"Dr. Jamie Marich educates us about dissociation from her personal experience combined with her extensive professional work. She helps us realize that to one extent or another we all use dissociation as a mechanism for coping with stress, trauma, and pain. With her example, readers will be inspired to recognize and accept without shame their own dissociative experiences and to seek support from knowledgeable guides. The book begins with an informative glossary of terms related to the subject of dissociation and ends with an extensive resource section that references podcasts, books, apps, and other helpful recovery tools. Between these bookends, the reader is treated to a guided and instructive tour of the territory associated with dissociation. A must-read for any clinician working with trauma, as well as anyone who experiences dissociation or who has a relationship with someone who does."

—PAUL FOXMAN, PhD, author of *Dancing with Fear*

"*Dissociation Made Simple* has taken my understanding as a trauma-informed somatic therapist to a whole new level. Rather than striving for an integration of the parts to achieve healing, author Jamie Marich says the goal should be deep listening to and interacting with the parts involved in settling destructive impulses. This book will turn you inside out and sideways. Bravo to Jamie Marich—a truly exciting and moving endeavor."

—STEPHANIE CITRON, PhD, clinical psychologist and trainer

"Dr. Marich writes with compassion and understanding about a topic so many still do not understand. She instructs readers how to recast their unique experiences with dissociation as the superpower it is. Like her other works, *Dissociation Made Simple* will become a well-worn guidebook for its mix of theory, practice, and personal narrative leading to a more dissociation-informed population."

—AARON SANDERS, director of GARAGE and Founder of *72 Hour Hold*

"I am always amazed by and appreciative of Dr. Jamie Marich's work, and she has done it again with *Dissociation Made Simple*. Her incredible lived experience paired with her immense professional knowledge; her open, vulnerable, and direct writing style; and her willingness to dissect complex ideas and make them 'simple,' is such a gift. I highly recommend this book to professionals and laypeople alike interested in learning more about a topic that impacts so many of us."

—MARISSA GHAVAMI, founder and artistic director of Healing TREE (Trauma Resources, Education & Entertainment)

"This book written so carefully and with high attention gives a fantastic understanding of dissociation through shared lived experiences—at a deep, core level. As a clinical psychologist and psychotherapist with years of experience, this book helped me to understand that there is more to learn. Dr. Jamie Marich makes it simple for us professionals and for all people who experience dissociation to understand what we should know and how we should approach and work from now on."

—ADELINA PJETRA, CEO and founder of Mental Health Albania

"A refreshing and respectful exploration of dissociation based on the voices of sixty others. Dr. Marich breaks the myths, reduces the stigma, and affirms and authentically explores the diversity of experience. She also provides tools and questions for the reader to explore their own experience of dissociation and its roots (e.g., trauma, cultural oppression, unquestioned-systemic power, etc.). It was hard to put the book down, as I so appreciated the accessible wisdom within."

—SUE GENEST, MSc. RCC, CCC, founder and director of Life Journeys Counselling and Training, Inc.

"*Dissociation Made Simple* is written in Dr. Marich's usual way—very personal, vulnerable, provocative, and forceful. Marich challenges some of my own preconceived ideas and paradigms and pushes the boundaries of what we think we know. In my mind, that's the only way we grow, so for that and many other reasons, I am very grateful for Dr. Marich for her work."

—DAN GRIFFIN, author of *A Man's Way through Relationships*

"No-nonsense, jargon-free, accessible, threaded through with Jamie Marich's own experience, *Dissociation Made Simple* is the book for anyone, therapist or client, who wants to know what dissociation feels like on the inside and therefore how best to work with it."

—MARK BRAYNE, former BBC foreign correspondent and founder of *EMDR Focus*

"Whether you are an individual living with a dissociative disorder or a mental health professional helping clients with dissociation, this book is your guide to destigmatizing dissociation, embracing dissociative parts, and reshaping the way you have perceived dissociation."

—ROTEM BREYER, MEd, LPC, founder of *The Art and Science of EMDR*

"Insightful, stigma-smashing, and lovingly well-informed, this book . . . masters beautifully what our field should have done all along: honor and amplify the voices of those with lived experience."

—TYNDAL E. SCHREINER, MA, LPC, blogger and social media educator

Dissociation Made Simple

A STIGMA-FREE GUIDE TO EMBRACING YOUR DISSOCIATIVE MIND AND NAVIGATING DAILY LIFE

JAMIE MARICH, PHD

FOREWORD BY JAIME POLLACK, MED, ITDS

North Atlantic Books

Huichin, unceded Ohlone land
aka Berkeley, California

Published by
North Atlantic Books
Huichin, unceded Ohlone land
aka Berkeley, California

"Window of Tolerance" illustration by Manal Al-Dabbagh
Other interior illustrations by Irene Rodriguez and Pungki Siregar
Cover illustration © anmark via Getty Images
Cover design by Amanda Weiss
Book design by Happenstance Type-O-Rama

Printed in the United States of America

Dissociation Made Simple: A Stigma-Free Guide to Embracing Your Dissociative Mind and Navigating Daily Life is sponsored and published by North Atlantic Books, an educational nonprofit based in the unceded Ohlone land Huichin (*aka* Berkeley, CA) that collaborates with partners to develop cross-cultural perspectives; nurture holistic views of art, science, the humanities, and healing; and seed personal and global transformation by publishing work on the relationship of body, spirit, and nature.

North Atlantic Books' publications are distributed to the US trade and internationally by Penguin Random House Publisher Services. For further information, visit our website at www.northatlantic books.com.

Library of Congress Cataloging-in-Publication Data

Names: Marich, Jamie, author.
Title: Dissociation made simple : a stigma-free guide to embracing your
   dissociative mind and navigating daily life / Jamie Marich.
Description: Huichin, unceded Ohlone land aka Berkeley, California : North
   Atlantic Books, [2022] | Includes bibliographical references and index.
Identifiers: LCCN 2022015623 (print) | LCCN 2022015624 (ebook) | ISBN
   9781623177218 (trade paperback) | ISBN 9781623177225 (ebook)
Subjects: LCSH: Dissociation (Psychology)
Classification: LCC RC553.D5 M32 2022 (print) | LCC RC553.D5 (ebook) |
   DDC 616.85/23—dc23/eng/20220831
LC record available at https://lccn.loc.gov/2022015623
LC ebook record available at https://lccn.loc.gov/2022015624

1 2 3 4 5 6 7 8 9 KPC 28 27 26 25 24 23

For my "girls"—Four, Nine, and Nineteen

Thank you for taking the ride with me!

Contents

Acknowledgments

To Shayna Keyles and the entire team at North Atlantic Books for allowing me to write the book that I wanted and needed to write at this time in my life ...

To everyone in my professional circles, especially those beautiful souls on the Institute for Creative Mindfulness team, who have supported me every step of the way in being out and vocal about my lived experience as a person with a dissociative disorder ...

To my community of fellow individuals who identify as plurals and/or survivors who are fighting the good fight to advocate for more equitable and human treatment of people everywhere ...

To each and every contributor whose wisdom appears in *Dissociation Made Simple*—I am forever changed by your example and your courage. I am so happy that many of you are in my life beyond this book, and that many of you have come into my life because of this book. May our conversations continue ...

To my inner circle of friends and loved ones who accept Jamie and all her parts exactly as they are. As I/we have prepared this book, special loving gratitude is extended to Allison Bugzavich, Dharl Chintan, Jeremy Sussel, Brendan and Ethan Reiter, Holly Petro, Sam Ore, Stacy Piccolo, Matt Vansuch, Richard Bruxvoort Colligan, and my dear teacher Christine Valters Paintner ...

We use the ellipsis (...) to represent that no English words can possibly do justice to describing the depth of our gratefulness, and to indicate that we wish for each and every collaboration noted here to continue on indefinitely. Only through conversations, collaboration, and connection will we bring about the change that is needed in our own lives and for the healing of the world entire. Thank you, dear friends, for joining us in this process.

Glossary of Terms

Many contributors to this book project shared that when they first learned about dissociation, the terminology around dissociation felt confusing and difficult to understand. While all of these terms are fully explored in the book, we've provided this glossary here for you at the beginning as a quick reference if you are reading and suddenly find yourself lost about the meaning of a term. We hope that you find this glossary tool helpful in your journey of discovery throughout this book. These definitions are not comprehensive and are meant only to be a starting point. You may come up with definitions after reading further that make more sense to you in your process.

addiction: derives from the Latin *addictus*, meaning "to be fixated on" or "favoring something"; in general, continuing to consume a substance or engage in a behavior that is reinforcing even when there is evidence of pain and consequences

Addiction as Dissociation model: developed by Adam O'Brien and Jamie Marich, the model posits that when children grow up in traumatizing, invalidating, or high-stress environments, the natural tendencies we have as humans to dissociate in order to get our needs met and protect ourselves happen so frequently that our systems bond to this dissociative experience. At a later point in life when chemicals or other reinforcing behaviors are introduced into our life as possibilities, the chemical impact enhances the potency of an already familiar experience

alter: comes from the Freudian term alter ego; refers to a part perceiving themselves as a separate entity, often taking control of the system; can show up in Dissociative Identity Disorder and certain forms of Otherwise Specified Dissociative Disorder

amnesia: blocking out time or memory/recollection of something having occurred or a part even existing; can present in various degrees within dissociative disorders

co-conscious: two or more parts/alters sharing consciousness at the same time (i.e., not blacking out, "going away," etc.)

core self: a term sometimes used by people with dissociative systems to refer to the primary or presenting self; not everyone with a dissociative system necessarily identifies as having a core self

dissociation: comes from a Latin root word, *dissociātiō*, meaning "to sever" or "to separate"; in clinical understanding, dissociation is the inherent human tendency to sever from the present moment when it becomes unpleasant or overwhelming. Dissociation can also refer to severed or separated aspects of self

ego state: generally refers to aspects of the personality based in unresolved material (e.g., the frightened child); although these ego states can feel separate and distinct, they do not necessarily contain the degree of fragmentation that would be required for a part to be considered a dissociative alter

fragmentation: a term for separation or more rigid splitting off of ego states or alters; sometimes referred to as "splitting"

fronting: refers to whichever part or alter appears to be in charge or speaking for the system at any given time; sometimes called "being out front"

grounding: using all available senses and all available experiences to remain in or return to the present moment

host: another older term for the core self or primary adult or presenting personality in a person with Dissociative Identity Disorder; not everyone with DID identifies a host body

hypnosis: generally a brain state where a person achieves heightened focus and concentration and is more open to suggestion; often conflated with dissociation although it is a separate construct

introject: based on a term from Gestalt therapy, can refer to parts that are intruding with the process of the core self or the entire system, and sometimes seem to align with a perpetrator or an abusive figure

littles: a colloquial term among people with Dissociative Identity Disorder or other dissociative disorders used to refer to the youngest parts in the system, those with child-like qualities

mindfulness: the practice of returning to the present moment or noticing whatever is in the present moment, without judgment

parts: a general term used in the psychological and helping professions that can refer to many different things. Parts is the most generic term possible that can be used to describe aspects, sides, or facets of self that do not necessarily represent the presence of another ego state. Some people even conceptualize their parts as the various roles they occupy in life: for instance, mother, teacher, friend, client, bowler, social justice advocate, etc.

perpetrator-identifying part: denotes a part that either takes on the qualities of a perpetrator or abuser, or aligns/takes the side in some way of the perpetrator or abuser

plural (or plurality): a colloquial term for people with dissociative disorders that identify having a system with many parts or alters; people with Dissociative Identity Disorder and other dissociative disorders can identify as being plural

psychosis: comes from the Greek *psyche*, meaning "animation of life"; typically identified by reality testing in the form of delusions and hallucinations

switching: a movement back and forth between different parts or aspects that are fronting; some people switch often and rapidly, some very subtly or not at all

trance: a state of semiconsciousness in which a person is not fully responsive to external stimulation; can be a state that is associated with many things, like dissociation, hypnosis, or meditation

trauma: comes from the Greek word meaning "wound"; in the human services, relates to any unhealed wound (physical, emotional, psychological, sexual, or spiritual in nature). Unhealed trauma can manifest as a variety of clinical diagnoses in the Diagnostic and Statistical Manual of Mental Disorders (DSM)

Foreword

It has been such an honor to get to know Dr. Jamie Marich—first as a colleague, whom I respected and admired, and now as a friend. As founder of An Infinite Mind (AIM), an international nonprofit organization that supports people living with dissociation and dissociative identities, I have met many people who live with, treat, and/or support others with dissociation. I am also a person living with dissociation and DID. So, I have firsthand experience with the subject. With all those factors considered, I can say that Jamie is truly a gift to this community.

When she asked me to both lend my voice to this project and write the foreword for the book, there wasn't a moment of hesitation. I have read several of her published books and have always been impressed with her ability to really connect with the reader on a personal and professional level. When we met in person at the annual Healing Together conference that AIM organizes, I found her to be as engaging, sincere, passionate, and dedicated as her books suggest.

I have had the privilege to get a glimpse of all the wonderful, different, and special parts that make up Jamie. I am excited she has now chosen to share those with all of you. Her book combines viewpoints from her personal experience and from her clinical work as a therapist and trainer in the field.

This book is a much-needed blend of science and first-person accounts. It includes all voices in the ongoing conversation including Indigenous and other marginalized populations, clinicians, and supporters. The combination of Western and Eastern views on dissociation help readers see it as something so natural that it leads them to wonder if dissociation should be considered a disorder at all.

In the book, everyone's unique experiences are accepted and valued. There are no boxes one must fit into. Instead, readers are given the choice to choose the wording that best fits them. They can explore the different healing options, as the journey is never one-size-fits-all.

This book is the voice of the community it serves. It shows how dissociation impacts everyone similarly yet also differently. As one of the contributors so perfectly put it, "I am typical of someone with DID, but I am not stereotypical."

One of my frustrations with reading self-help books is the lingering feeling of, "Thank you for the information. But, now what do I do with it?" Jamie was proactive in answering that type of question. At the end of every chapter, readers will find activities and questions to support their learning, deepen their understanding, and continue the conversation with their therapists. Grounding supports are also weaved throughout the book, and readers are encouraged to use them as needed.

Throughout the pages, readers will find powerful metaphors and new perspectives. One of my personal favorites was viewing dissociation like a prism. It shines many different and beautiful colors when light hits it. I learned the power of one word: *enough*. The idea of feeling safe was something I couldn't feel. However, there are places in my life where I feel safe enough.

As Jamie so beautifully sums up, it is the hope of this book to normalize trauma responses and dissociation so people will gain the same level of compassion and understanding when they say they have DID as when they say they have PTSD. I believe she has done just that!

—JAIME POLLACK, MEd, ITDS, founder and
director of An Infinite Mind

Introduction

Dissociation Is Not a Dirty Word

The cosmos are also within us.
—CARL SAGAN

When I was about nine years old, the abusive figure that loomed largest in my life would regularly say, "Jamie, you look like you've been beaned in the head with a fast ball."

It's true, I wandered through life dazed and confused, as if I had just been walloped in the head with a monster pitch. Although I was never hit in the head with an actual baseball, this description still rang fairly accurate. Only that something that clobbered me was persistent, developmental trauma. And unlike in real baseball, there was no trainer to attend to me. I had to fend for myself, and this uncanny ability I developed to zone out was always there to help me.

The world of daydream and fantasy felt so much more appealing and yes, so much safer than the reality into which I was born and raised. So, it became very difficult to pay attention and stay present with whatever I was supposed to be doing at any given time. Once, I fell down a set of stairs on a junior high field trip to a museum in a nearby city, and my mother took me to the ER to get my head checked out later that evening.

"Jamie was probably off in her own world and not paying attention again," she told the attending physician.

Physically, my head was fine, and they sent me home that night.

Emotionally, I was only just beginning to see the evidence of how much this thing I later learned is called *dissociation* dominated my life.

My head was anything but fine.

Dissociation and the Human Experience

Dissociation is a normal part of the human experience, especially when we grow up chronically exposed to trauma and stress. Or when we are born into an environment where we feel misunderstood, marginalized, or otherwise chastised for living our fullest expression of ourselves. Yet dissociation remains one of the most misunderstood phenomena in both the mental health field and in society at large. We've gotten more savvy about understanding trauma, which can generally be defined as any unhealed human wound. These wounds can be emotional, physical, sexual, spiritual, somatic, financial, existential, or they can exist in any combination. The English word *trauma* comes from the Greek word *traumatikōs* meaning "wound."

You may even have heard the phrase *trauma-informed* used to describe care within a system. To be truly trauma-informed, or equipped to deal with the wide array of human wounding, we must become dissociation-informed as well because trauma and dissociation go hand in hand. Trauma survivors rely on some degree of dissociation in order to cope with and navigate life. Citing the wisdom of Amy Wagner, a colleague who lives with a dissociative experience of life, "If trauma is walking through the door of your clinic, dissociation is parking the car." You'll learn more about Amy's experience later in this book.

In larger society, the word *dissociation* is fortunately coming into wider use. Yet if the public knows anything about the clinical manifestations of dissociation, it's most likely the old label of *Multiple Personality Disorder*. And media portrayal of Multiple Personality Disorder in the era of earlier *Diagnostic and Statistical Manuals (DSM),* and now the portrayal of what is presently called Dissociative Identity Disorder (DID), is typically sensationalized, inaccurate, or both. Only the most extreme cases tend to be highlighted in all forms of media—including the popularity of DID on social media platforms like TikTok—which heightens the stigma, promotes the spread of misinformation, and can ultimately make people afraid of dissociation. As many contributors to this book pointed out, even the more responsible portrayals of dissociative disorders in media are still highly problematic because they can focus on the most dramatic aspects of dissociative disorders, like *switching* between parts or alters on a regular basis. As Jaime Pollack, a woman living with DID and founder of the revolutionary organization An Infinite Mind pointed out in an interview with me, "I think most people would be surprised to see how boring and routine my life really is."

Yes, you may be frightened when you realize that dissociation applies to you, just as so many clinicians out there can be fearful of addressing it with you. Yet the aim of this book is to share more stories like Jaime's so that we can all be less afraid of how dissociation shows up in the human experience. Because at the end of the day, even though dissociation can cause its share of problems individually and at the societal level, our ability as humans to dissociate truly is a superpower—this recurring theme popped out more than any others in conducting interviews with sixty-one contributors for this book. Another major theme that emerged from interviewing contributors for this book project is that *dissociation is not a dirty word.* I know of several clinicians who hear the word *dissociation,* or see signs of it in their office, and automatically think it's a problem. While dissociation, or specifically the traumatic roots of it, can cause problems in daily living or in societal systems—problems that need to be addressed—dissociation is the skill that has allowed so many of us to survive and, in many ways, to thrive.

I write this book primarily for the general public and people struggling with mental health who may have heard the word *dissociation* in reference to themselves. Maybe you saw the popular meme floating around at the beginning of the COVID-19 pandemic that touted: "Some of you lack the dissociative skills to survive the apocalypse, and it shows," and inside said to yourself . . . um, that's me! Perhaps you've even received a formal diagnosis or are working with a therapist on another mental health issue and they mentioned that dissociation or *parts* may be a factor in your case.

You may be the loved one of someone with a dissociative disorder or someone navigating complex trauma recovery, and reading this book is an effort to better support the person you care about. If you are a therapist reading this book, you likely picked it up to better understand what's going on with your clients. You may even be a teacher, a coach, or another professional who is reading this book with a similar intention of learning how to better help the people you serve. Yet I challenge you to consider that to truly do that, you must first do some deep digging on how dissociation manifests in your own life. Engaging in this personal work is definitely not easy, yet it's one of the surest ways to "make simple" (or at least, *simpler*) the process of understanding dissociation, embracing it, and navigating its manifestations in daily life.

Whatever led you to pick up a copy of this book, I recognize that exploring your own relationship with dissociation can feel frightening. I also know from personal experience that *not* engaging in this exploration and healing can be an even greater risk. At the very least, you may remain further *dissociated* from the life you deserve to be living.

What Does Dissociation *Even Mean?*

You may be asking yourself this question or something similar right now, after the opening passage. If you've been in therapy before or currently are in therapy, your provider may or may not have been able to explain it to you in a way that makes any kind of sense. If you're a therapist, you may have read several books and gone to many clinical trainings and still find yourself stumped. That's how I felt, even as a woman with a diagnosed dissociative disorder, when I attended my first EMDR (Eye Movement Desensitization and Reprocessing) Therapy training and listened to a well-known expert speak on dissociation. I left scratching my head and wondering what I had just listened to. Similarly, whenever I tried to read many of the classically clinical books in the field on dissociation, I would either throw them down in frustration or struggle to get through them.

"We're not a science project!" I would cry in protest.

And my head would scramble even further when I saw myself and others like me turned into one.

The meanings and implications of dissociation are the first items we explore in this book (chapter 1), so please know that much more depth will follow. For now, consider this basic working definition: *Dissociation* comes from a Latin root, *dissociātiō*, meaning "to sever" or "to separate." As people we can sever from the present moment when that reality becomes overwhelming or unpleasant, or we can experience a profound separation within our core self when we are unable to process or fully integrate an experience. My goal is to empower you with knowledge from a variety of perspectives to best understand dissociation and the various ways it can show up in you and how you relate to the world. Through this knowledge base, we will cover some basic skills that you can learn to keep yourself safe enough and grounded for the healing journey ahead (chapter 2). These are skills that can be done on your own, or together with any professional therapy you are receiving. Guidelines for keeping yourself as safe as possible are offered throughout the book, and every chapter features a "Questions to Ask My Therapist or Psychiatrist" section to help you best self-advocate.

The book features three guided exercises, *Parts Mapping* (chapter 4), *The Dissociative Profile* (chapter 5), and *Parts Scene Work* (chapter 5). Although best done together with a therapist or other professional, all of these exercises can be explored on one's own as long as the safety precautions covered in this introduction and chapter 2 are respected. You are *not* required to have a clinical diagnosis of a dissociative disorder or other mental health concern to benefit from these exercises. Because dissociation is such a regular part of the human experience, we can all benefit from exploring our relationships with the ways we dissociate. This message constitutes a core theme of the book.

We all *sever* from the present moment in one way or another. Sometimes it's not problematic, and other times it is. This book gives you the tools to make that determination for yourself. Moreover, we all have *parts* of self. You do not have to carry a diagnosis of Dissociative Identity Disorder (DID) in order to relate to having an *inner child* or a part that is easily angered. If you struggle with addiction or other behavioral compulsions, you may feel like there is a part of you that wants to be sober, and another part that wants to keep acting out. You may use the word *compartmentalize* quite often in describing your life and how you are able to negotiate the value differences between your work life and your family life. Notice that the word *part* is the central root of this word frequently used in our modern times. Parts work is truly for all of us.

Normalizing dissociation is a huge aspect of how we change the conversation around it in order to combat the myths and misconceptions. One such myth is that people with dissociative disorders are so unstable, they will never be able to live a functional and thriving life. Indeed, most people with dissociative disorders, even Dissociative Identity Disorder, are high functioning. The dissociative mind develops many skills, and one of these is an ability to hide things well. Another gift can be the ability to use dissociative functions adaptively for survival. Yet in other areas of life, we may be experiencing a great deal of exhaustion, distress, and shame—which can bring us to therapy in the first place. And too often we are met with professionals who either don't know how to handle us, *or* professionals who don't even believe that dissociation is real.

Choosing a mental health provider who understands dissociation and its intricacies can be imperative to your success in meeting your goals for healing.

In chapter 6 we cover best practices for treatment of trauma-related dissociation and dissociative disorders. This chapter includes guidelines on how best to choose a therapist, and what qualities to look for in other healing professionals. The applicability of many trauma-focused therapies in working with trauma-related dissociation, specifically dissociative disorders, is presented for your information in order to make informed choices. Trauma-informed and trauma-focused care must, above anything else, work with your right to informed and empowered choice.

People with dissociative disorders have grown used to doing a significant amount of advocating for ourselves. This imperative sadly becomes necessary when many professionals feel like they are in over their heads when working with us. Chapter 7 and the conclusion that follows address the important role of advocacy in reducing stigma. We discuss how people can advocate for themselves, and how survivors of trauma—working together with professionals—can create a paradigm shift around trauma and dissociation in society.

These final chapters also give crucial guidance about how to sensitively handle the *coming out* process. You may only associate *coming out* as a phrase that relates to sexuality or gender identity, yet it is plenty relevant as a concept in mental health. People constantly worry about folks finding out about the fullness of their diagnosis and what this may mean for their standing in the community, for their career, and for their reputation. Such concerns are not unique to dissociative disorders, yet they can feel especially brutal for people with dissociative disorders because so much misunderstanding abounds. The book also contains two appendices specifically for helping professionals and for loved ones of people with dissociative disorders and complex trauma. We ask you to consult these sections only *after* you have read and worked through the other content in the book, in order to get the most out of what they can offer.

The *expressive arts,* a term used to refer to the multimodal (e.g., different practices like making art, dancing, drumming, singing, writing) and intermodal (e.g., working with several forms at once or acknowledging their interplay), is incorporated throughout *Dissociation Made Simple.* My friend and collaborator Irene Rodriguez created beautiful illustrations to accompany each chapter, assisted by her colleague Pungki Siregar. You are free to color these and be creative with them, especially if you struggle with grounding and find this kind of expressive work with coloring to be helpful. For many of us with dissociative experiences of life (i.e., dissociative disorders or dissociative identities), these nonlinear and verbal-optional practices are the way we make sense of the world and best express ourselves.

Although the professional "Dr. Jamie" is a Registered Expressive Arts Therapist and educator, our passion for sharing the expressive arts with you comes from a much more personal place. Throughout our childhood, the expressive arts, especially dancing, playing and listening to music, creative writing, and theater saved us. They gave us an outlet for being able to process what was happening in our inner world most of the time in ways that were not destructive. And when I (Jamie) presented for my own healing work with professionals in my early twenties, this extensive engagement with expressive practices made us more willing to open up emotionally to do the work that I/we needed to do in order to heal. As I explain in the next section and develop in several places throughout the book, people who identify as having dissociative experiences of life may be very fluid with their pronouns or have very specific requests for you about which pronouns they use and how they identify as navigators of the world.

Bridging the Personal and the Professional

Outside of the field, when I tell people that I have a dissociative disorder, I am usually met with, "What does that mean?"

The easiest explanation can sound something like, "You've heard of Multiple Personality Disorder, right? Well it's not called that anymore, and even if it were, I have a milder form of it. All of my parts are aware of each other's existence and we don't block out time as adults, even though there are chunks of our childhood that we don't remember."

Then people can look at me wondering if I'm Sybil, or if like Edward Norton's character Aaron Stampler in *Primal Fear*, I'm just faking it for attention or as an excuse for bad behavior.

To set the record straight, I am not Sybil.

This statement is referencing the 1976 movie starring Sally Field, based on the book by Flora Rheta Schreiber. The book, while initially presented as nonfiction, was later exposed to be highly fictionalized and exploitative. Yet the damage of the *Sybil* phenomenon permeated the mental health field and larger society. At least five other contributors to this book also stated, very directly, "I am not Sybil" in their interviews, and many more referenced the film and book as having done much harm to how people who experience dissociation are received.

I am out in all areas of my life as a bisexual woman, and I've also been very candid about my struggles with addiction since entering the helping professions. Yet nothing filled me with the terror of this coming out quite like coming out as someone living with dissociative experiences, because I know how terrible my colleagues can be about all things dissociative disorders and dissociation. Since formally entering the clinical field in 2004, I've heard dissociation talked about with such negation ("It doesn't even exist," or "They're making it all up"), fear ("I'm just afraid I'm not going to be able to bring them back," "I don't want to destabilize them"), or dismissal ("I won't offer people the treatment I do if they score above a certain number on the screening tool I give"). For years, I would sit back at conferences, even in the EMDR community to which I belong and listen to people—even the "experts"—talk about dissociation in a way that concerned me. When attending many of these expert dissociation presentations at a variety of conferences, I feel like the presenters—while knowledgeable—are usually talking *about* people like me instead of presenting with a personal sense of connection to the material. The heart and soul has been missing in so much professional content.

For years my colleagues asked me when I was going to put together a training on dissociation, specifically for EMDR therapists. I knew that I didn't want to be one more presenter citing slide after slide of other people's research, nor did I want to be up there talking in code. In other words, I didn't want to play off my lived experience as something *the literature said.* While the two often coincide, I felt it would be disrespectful to my larger community of people struggling with dissociative disorders and identities to continue in that vein. While I've not exactly hidden the fact that I've struggled with dissociation in previous writing (including my first book, *EMDR Made Simple,* published in 2011), in 2018 I made the decision to come out—fully and unapologetically— as a woman in recovery from a dissociative disorder. In doing that, I experienced a great sense of liberation to train about, to speak on, and to write about dissociation in a way that represents the paradigm shift I believe we need to change the conversation and shatter stigma.

So what happened in 2018 to cause the shift? Part of the context is that I was already an established author and teacher in this field, which emboldened me with a sense of, "If they're not going to listen to me after all this time because I have a dissociative mind, they're probably not going to be the type who will listen to my voice anyway." Honestly, I felt similarly when I got my nose pierced in 2014, something I'd always wanted to do but was afraid of how it might reflect on me professionally. There is a joy that opens up in life when we can start to care less about what others think. I believe that if more of us can learn to do this through our own healing journeys, we can move many of the barriers that I discuss throughout the book to dissociation—and all mental health concerns—being taken seriously.

More significantly, at the end of 2017 one of my greatest fears came true—my ex-husband tried to use my dissociative disorder against me in a very brutal way. One of my parts (Nine) holds our tendencies to self-injure and self-destruct, something that developed when we were chronologically nine. The marriage didn't stand a chance of surviving, the more my system worked on allowing Jamie to present as her truest self in the world. That, coupled with the triggering fallout we experienced after the 2016 U.S. presidential election, caused a re-emergence of self-injury, both internal and external. Our ex-spouse caught one of these episodes on video without us knowing, and then posted it online in an attempt to shame me and to discredit my work. When he tried and failed, and I experienced a tremendous amount of support from my friends and the healing team around me, I knew that I had nothing to be afraid of anymore and here I am . . . sharing candidly on how we experience the world.

As your guide through the material in this book, I am an advocate, a clinical professional and educator, and a survivor of my own complex trauma, most of which was religious in nature. My experience with the phenomenon of dissociation is an intimate one—I've been doing it most of my life in response to trauma and stress, and in 2004 my first trauma-focused therapist formally diagnosed me with Dissociative Disorder, Not Otherwise Specified (NOS). In the currently updated DSM-5, my condition would be best described as an Otherwise Specified Dissociative Disorder (OSDD) Type 1, although I intimately relate to those who have DID and during some seasons of my life feel more connection to that diagnosis. OSDD Type 1 is considered closest to DID, and we discuss these descriptors more fully in chapter 1.

My system is composed of separate and distinct parts that are co-conscious: aware of each other's existence and fully aware of what the other parts are doing or saying at any given time. You will learn about us more throughout the book and how we, and others like us, are more than just our diagnoses. We are Four-, Nine-, and Nineteen-year-old versions of Jamie, which are aligned with the chronological ages when we experienced major trauma and upheaval in our system. Until recently, Jamie chose not to assign names to the other parts and simply calls them *Four*, *Nine*, and *Nineteen* (which many people with dissociative disorders will do), reflecting that we are all Jamie, just Jamie at differently frozen states in her development. We are not separate and distinct people; we are part of a larger system that honors Jamie's inherent wholeness. We continue to help her navigate daily life through stressful terrains filled with the land mines that are potential trauma triggers. Often these triggers create a significant sense of *derealization,* or leaving us to question whether something is truly happening in the tangible world, or just being experienced in our mind. For many survivors of trauma with dissociative expressions, what happens in the inner world is just as real as how others might experience the outer world, and managing these expressions can be one of the most challenging parts of living with a dissociative disorder.

We, the parts, are "in the car" with Jamie as her presently adult self driving the car. When one of us is struggling or working through a stressful life event rooted in some past trauma, we do everything to get her attention so that it becomes hard for her to drive. And she then has to stop to take care of herself and all of us, because we are all in relationship with each other. When one of us is suffering, the entire system can feel it. As an example, one of Jamie's great traumatic losses and resulting abuses happened when she was chronologically nineteen. At the time of this writing, Four (whom we sometimes call Lucy) can feel most affected by that memory's imprint in our system because it was Four that first experienced emotional abandonment as a template for receiving the world.

The parts that compose our system do not experience significant amnestic blackouts that might be more associated with the DID diagnosis. So the adult Jamie driving the car remains the driver even though the others may make it difficult to drive. In DID, the other parts may fully take over the wheel. In our system, we've learned to operate in good communication with each other as a result of over twenty years of healing experiences. The car is our chosen metaphor for describing our system to others, yet as we will discuss in chapter 5, there are numerous metaphors that you can explore to help you better understand and work with your system. And how we describe our system is just one example of how a system may be experienced. Every contributor to this book with an identified system had something to say about how their system formed, exists, and lives, and we are excited to share these insights with you throughout the book. If Jamie's description of how her parts interplay doesn't fully resonate with you, please keep reading; you will likely find other voices in this book that will.

Parts and systems can also be more than just age representations of ego states. They may also contain different aspects of the totality that are either working together—or causing disruption if they are not being sufficiently seen. For me/us, this plays out in the Dr. Jamie/Jamie battle. When I/we give a training or write an article or book, "Dr. Jamie" and all her wisdom are usually out front doing the work, yet we are informed by the experiences of Jamie's entire system. Sometimes, Jamie (the personal system that includes all of the parts and Jamie's nonprofessional adult self) does not let Dr. Jamie speak or *front*, a term sometimes used in the dissociative disorders community. When we feel it's important that people, especially professionals, hear us from a very raw place, Jamie takes over. We've consciously decided to let that more personal voice navigate the journey of this book, and we're delighted that contributors who have agreed to be interviewed are willing to share from that personal space too.

In this book we write with a mixture of our personal and professional voice, because both are equally important parts that compose the total self. Sometimes the subject *I* is used in my writing, other times I lean into the subject *we*, (e.g., "In this chapter, we will cover the fundamentals of parts work"). Many individuals with a high level of distinction in their systems will use the singular *we* pronoun in their discourse, and this applies to us too. Issues around pronouns are covered more fully in chapter 5. For many years, I noticed my tendency to refer to ourselves as *we*, and adult Jamie made a conscious effort to correct it, especially in the name of professional credibility. Now, we've learned to embrace our sense of *we*-ness, or plurality, and write from that place.

Can Understanding Dissociation Really Be Made Simple?

With everything I've presented so far, you may be wondering if understanding dissociation can ever be *made simple*. I am the first to admit that the title of this book may be an oxymoron, especially because what we call dissociation can be so many things. And I also admit that nothing infuriates me more in my field than when trainers try to reduce working with dissociation down to "5 Easy Steps," or promise that you can attain full mastery in a weekend workshop. As Katarina Felicia Lundgren, a brilliant Swedish equine therapist with DID who shared her lived experience for this book expressed, "the need to make me *simpler* is just going to hurt more."

I resonate a great deal with her comments, and they represent a major reason I struggled with how best to title this book. I ultimately chose *Dissociation Made Simple* as the main title because I already wrote two other "made simple" books—*EMDR Made Simple* in 2011 and *Trauma Made Simple* in 2014. My intention with this book is to activate the same voice I used for the two earlier books and thus help alleviate the fear that some clinicians experience around these topics. In the two previous books, I also gave clinicians ideas for how to work within the rather dysfunctional mental health systems of North America, while also issuing calls to action for how we can bring about change. With *Dissociation Made Simple,* which is written for an even wider audience and with even stronger use of my own lived experience, I also hope to defuse the land mines of fear that can make us tread so lightly that we become afraid of our own shadows. If a savvy title like *Dissociation Made Simple* makes it more likely that people will pick this book up in the first place to engage in the important work of navigating their own fears, then I am okay with keeping the title.

Another point is one that I made in the introduction of *EMDR Made Simple* over a decade ago, and it is also relevant here: the best way to make understanding something simple is to embrace its complexity. As I tell my students, I was an English teacher and expressive artist long before I became a therapist, and I approach this material with the heart of someone steeped in the humanities, not the hard sciences. So I very often use etymology, or digging into the root of a word's origin in the English language, to help us better understand it clinically. The word *complex* first surfaced in 1652 (a Latin derivation) meaning "composed of several parts." In 1715, an alternate usage emerged, with the word *complexity* meaning "something that is not easily analyzed."[1] Both of these definitions help us to see what is going on with dissociation. Whether it be a person's parts system or merely the acceptance that as a person, we are not just a body, just a mind, just a spirit—we are the totality of everything working together. In the brilliant teaching of Roger Vielle, an elder in the Blackfeet nation who contributed his experience for this book, "We are all our own universe within a universe."

For contributor Julian Jaramillo, an Ecuadorian psychotherapist trained in the Shamanic traditions of the Chocó people, dissociation is simply "a lack of relationship." When there is a breakdown in communication or a fissure between the different aspects of us working together and learning from each other, dissociation may be present. And once we notice that dissociation is present, we can challenge ourselves to reconnect with our inherent wholeness.

The 1715 definition offers an even more potent foundation for what we are trying to do in this book—recognizing that there is no easy formula or analysis for trying to work with dissociative minds. Speaking for my system and many like us who contributed to the book, we can get very upset when thought leaders in the field of dissociation try to put us into a box by giving inventories like the Dissociative Experiences Scale (DES) and the Multidimensional Inventory of Dissociation (MID) and believing they know us just by interpreting the results. We get even more upset when we hear that people feel they need one of these tools—which can be useful in the right contexts—to even know that they are dealing with a dissociative mind. While we also recognize these quantitative measures are important in proving to the field at large that dissociation and dissociative disorders are real, deep down many of us are resentful because our minds—which are inherently qualitative and limitless—are being reduced into the box of numbers and science.

And then there are the countless models and methods that now exist for doing "parts work" in the clinical professions. While myself and many of my fellow dissociative minds don't necessarily oppose these models and even use some of them ourselves as clinicians, what we resent is the idea that we can be reduced to a simple model like Internal Family Systems (IFS) or the Theory of Structural Dissociation. In the very candid expression of Heather (LS) Scarboro+, a nonbinary/transmasculine individual living with DID who also works as a clinician, "The language of IFS, as beautiful as it is for a basic groundwork for parts, really pisses DID folks off. . . . You're talking to me like my system fits into this long, multifaceted terminology about shit. There's a huge disconnect."

Indeed, a question that can make my blood boil is when my students, consultees, and readers ask me what model I use for parts work. My general answer is that I draw on aspects of all of them but that they all have their limitations, and truly understanding dissociation—especially its clinical manifestations like DID—involves recognizing that no one model can ever capture it all. Our inquiry must go beyond our field's tendency to put everything into tidy models and wrap them up with a bow that can be easily packaged as a training or book. Even I admit in writing this book that I am not going to teach you everything you need to know and if anyone ever promises you that they can, you're being lied to. To truly simplify your relationship with understanding dissociation, you must start by embracing the complex nature of human existence. In this book I encourage you to move beyond the inventories and the models and to accept the invitation into this deeper work. The phenomenological nature of this book will hopefully make this process simpler for us . . . simpler, but not easy.

Phenomenology: Celebrating Our Lived Experience

In her doctoral work, Dr. Jamie was trained as a phenomenologist and has published extensively using methodologies grounded in the philosophical approach of Moravian-German philosopher Edmund Husserl (1859–1938). From phenomenology, we get the term *lived experience*. Michael Crotty, a scholar who greatly influenced Dr. Jamie during her doctoral studies, explains that phenomenology rejects the Galilean notion that the human experience can be mathematically quantified. When we—Jamie's system—encountered this thinking in her doctoral studies, we rejoiced. We are neither anti-science nor anti–empirical research; we even acknowledge that many of our advocates needed to do the numbers and science to validate the reality of our minds and conditions for the scientific mainstream. Yet we firmly believe that numbers can never paint a complete picture of the human experience. We are more than just a series of numbers, measures, and statistical formulas.

Melissa Parker, a therapist with a diagnosis of DID based in New England who contributed her lived experience for this book, also feels very strongly about this disconnect.

She remarked, "Our stories have been written by those who don't know anything about us."

Melissa also describes the experience of being at academic and clinical conferences in our field and hearing many of the experts, including "those who others practically have shrines to in their office," say cold, uncaring, and insulting things about people with DID. She embraces the call to drown out these unhelpful voices with more voices of lived experience.

One of our collaborators who has become a true brother in this work is a therapist from upstate New York named Adam O'Brien. Although he is cited throughout this book as a personal contributor of lived experience and Jamie's coauthor of the Addiction as Dissociation model, for the time being, we will introduce you to Adam through this nugget of his wisdom. Says Adam, "You have to have a phenomenological or liberal arts approach or mindset before you can start touting science as a fact. The conscious brain ignoring emotional needs is where conflict exists. And quantitatively minded people have to realize how limiting research is when it does not include phenomenological approaches."

Dissociation Made Simple is a book that seeks to meet the need Adam describes. Even though neuroscience has been all the rage in the trauma-focused facets of the helping professions in recent years, we truly believe that reducing any psychological phenomenon to the neuroscience alone is limiting and, in the case of dissociation, misses the point. While I can acknowledge the importance of neuroscientific research in validating what we do and helping more science-minded clients understand that there can be good reasons behind why they behave the way that they do, I fear that our field's obsession with neuroscience has created its own form of dissociation. Emphasizing hard science alone can keep us dissociated from the other aspects of ourselves—namely the emotional and the spiritual (or whatever you may want to call that realm that surpasses rational understanding). Not to mention that keeping the focus solely on neuroscience cuts us off from millennia of Indigenous wisdom. According to Julian Jaramillo, "In traditional Shamanism the 'brain' doesn't quite exist, so there is no language to really name these things; they would speak about human experience as we name it, as we feel it."

When Julian, whom my own therapist Elizabeth Davis suggested I speak to for this book, conveyed this teaching in his interview with me, a jolt of energetic recognition passed through my body. Having felt more seen by Julian the Shaman than I ever felt by most of my peers at academic conferences, I knew that human experiences needed to be the feature of this book. I was, however, delighted that one member of the EMDR community who has made me feel very seen over the years, dissociative specialist Dr. Curt Rounazoin from Orange County, California, was willing to be interviewed for the book. Curt is that person in whose presence our Four part has always felt very safe, and this is a rarity in our professional world.

As Curt shared, reflecting on his forty-year career, "Most of the stuff I've learned how to do I've learned from my patients. I always tell my colleagues, 'Find a dissociative client and listen to them. That will make you a good therapist.'"

Contributor Wayne William Snellgrove, a member of the Fishing Lake First Nation in Saskatchewan, Canada and survivor of the Canadian residential school program that he refers to as genocide, offered powerful insight from his first Medicine Man: "The first ceremony that we need to learn is the ceremony of listening."

While *Dissociation Made Simple* does not discount the validity of empirical inquiry and neuroscience, it does boldly contend that these areas of inquiry are sorely insufficient if we truly want to understand and embrace dissociation. Like Curt and Wayne both suggest, we have to *listen* to people in order to best learn. Although we make some citations in the book for context, the voices of our sixty-one contributors constitute the primary evidence for the contentions made in *Dissociation Made Simple*. Instead of integrating clinical "case studies" into this book from clients Dr. Jamie served in a professional capacity, we've elected to involve the voices of people in our larger circles— some we know and others we've met through this book project—to share their lived experience. We invited many of our collaborators and professional contacts who we believe deeply understand the heart and soul of dissociative experiences to contribute, and several others came forward to speak about their journeys when we made news of this book public. Although the sharing is weaved in throughout the content of the book to provide the necessary color of lived experience, Dr. Jamie committed to conducting each interview with respect to phenomenological methodology in the event that she might publish these findings in more of a peer-reviewed forum later (assuming that our peers will have us).

Translated into plain language, this means that Dr. Jamie was inspired by the words and work of Edmund Husserl as she conducted the interviews, even making a conscious commitment to set aside her own experiences on dissociation to truly listen to what other people had to say. Because this is a book written for the general public and is not a pure research study, our presentation of what the interviews revealed is imparted not just through the lens of my lived experience, but rather through the lens of my system's experience. Yet I/we can honestly say that the experience of conducting these sixty-one interviews over a period of four months changed us—as a person/system, and as a therapist. So much of what I/we thought we knew about how to work with dissociation was challenged through listening very directly to people, and these experiences shared with us also lit a greater fire of enthusiasm in us to bring about change in the status quo of what it means to help people. I was even inspired through talking to our contributors to try out a few healing modalities that I had not yet considered for myself, including a guided psychedelic experience and engaging deeper in Native ceremonies.

As Husserl stated, "Phenomenology invites us to set aside all previous habits of thought, see through and break down the mental barriers which these habits have set along the horizons of our thinking . . . to learn to see what stands before our eyes."[2] In order to engage in this clear seeing, Dr. Jamie also composed what was called a semi-standardized interview informed by the protocols of Grant McCracken's *The Long Interview*.[3] This means that she asked every participant for this book project the same core questions after running through some basic grounding and safety procedures (e.g., letting contributors know they could stop or pause the interview at any time):

- What motivates you to take part in this interview process? As part of this introduction, please summarize any information about your background that you feel is most important for us to know.

- Based on your lived experience, how would you describe *dissociation* to someone if they asked you to explain it? How might you explain your specific diagnosis (if applicable)?

- Based on your lived experience, how would you describe what's happening in your brain and in your body during dissociative experiences?

- What are the most effective skills you've developed for yourself in order to keep yourself grounded or safe enough?

- If you identify as having a parts system, how would you describe your system?

- What, if anything, has been most effective for you so far in your process of healing? This may include professional treatment interventions or other nonclinical pursuits.

- You now have a platform to speak to all therapists, psychiatrists, and helping professionals everywhere. What best practices would you relay to them for working with people like you?

- What do you feel is needed to break the stigma around dissociation and other mental health disorders at a societal level?

- What are the positive aspects of living with a dissociative mind or dissociative experiences?

- What other experiences, from your perspective, might you want to share with others about any aspect of dissociation?

The experiences you will read about in this book flowed from this phenomenological process. Every contributor was given a chance to be interviewed under their legal name, their system's name, a pseudonym, or anonymously. All of the contributors were of adult age (over eighteen) at the time of the interview. Each contributor was given a chance to review how we wrote about their shared experience in the book's first draft, and they gave me clarifications and corrective feedback, which has been implemented in this finished product. While one could argue that these experiences yield content that is

more for adult readers, valuable insight can be gleaned for addressing dissociation in children. Many of the contributors identify child parts and most
speak of their connection to dissociation developing in childhood as a result
of early trauma.

Even though the majority of the contributors who came forward to offer
their lived experiences for the book were white women, seven of them directly
identified as queer, bisexual, or lesbian. Thirteen men came forward to
speak to me for the project. While a greater degree of diversity can always be
achieved in conducting projects such as this one, we are delighted that three
nonbinary folx, one person identifying as gender fluid (she/they pronouns),
eleven people of color, and several people from outside the United States (e.g.,
Canada, India, the United Kingdom, Ecuador, Sweden, and Ireland) agreed
to be interviewed for *Dissociation Made Simple*. Four of the contributors from
the United States and Canada identify as Native or Indigenous, and many
more are non-Native individuals who have responsibly engaged with Native
practices as part of their healing journey. There is a richness in these contributions that surpasses anything we may learn in Western psychology. In referencing contributors throughout the book, the identifiers about background
and demographics that a contributor provided will be noted, especially if
they are relevant to the experiences they described.

We are also delighted that, based on the public call for participation, so
many people came forward who do not distinctly have a diagnosed dissociative disorder. While twenty-seven contributors directly identified having a dissociative disorder either at the time of their interview or in the past (including
eighteen with DID), many different diagnoses are represented—most numer-
ously PTSD or complex PTSD with strong dissociative components. However,
depression, anxiety, substance use disorders, eating disorders, neurodivergence
(e.g., ADHD, autism spectrum), Borderline Personality Disorder, and schizoaffective disorder are also represented. Many people also decided to contribute
based on the level of dissociation they've experienced in navigating chronic
medical conditions or physical disability. And of course there are numerous
experiences shared about people who currently identify as having a dissociative disorder or a dissociative experience of life being misdiagnosed with so
many other things over the years—anything but the dissociation because their
providers were not willing or able to see the impact of trauma and dissociation.

The majority of individuals who were invited to or came forward to contribute interviews work as psychotherapists (thirty-nine in total), and several
others work in some other type of helping profession. This percentage may

feel like a limitation to some readers because there is generally an assumption that therapists naturally have a higher degree of insight about their own conditions. This assumption is far from the truth, in my experience. Moreover, the willingness of so many therapists to come forward who do have the dual insight of the personal and the professional was largely motivated by a common factor—feeling the need to speak up about their own stories in order to end stigma and create a change in the way that dissociative disorders are perceived. People of all professions and walks of life are impacted by dissociation, even therapists. Several other professions are also represented in our sample of contributors (e.g., lawyer, financial advisor, engineer, paramedic, executive manager, optician, preschool teacher, factory worker).

We hope that you relate to some aspect of yourself (or yourselves) in what many of our contributors share. And in this relation you may no longer feel so alone. Sharing lived experiences, we believe, is how we will truly bring about the change that is needed in the fields of the helping and healing professions, and ultimately in our world. We've hidden too long behind clinical jargon, myths, and fear of our body–mind systems and now—as so much of the world adapts to change—is as good a time as any to make this vital and necessary shift.

We Ask You to Take Care of Yourself

We hope you are intrigued by this opening challenge to explore how dissociation applies to you. Please know that whenever issues of trauma, abuse, and chronic mistreatment are discussed, the potential to be triggered is high. You may be reading and suddenly feel very activated, or you could be reading and suddenly find that you are struggling to pay attention, or feel like you are shutting down. Both can be valid responses that are covered more fully in our next chapter.

For now, I'm hoping that you will make a deal with us—that you will be gentle with yourself while reading this book and not push past those signals you are receiving. Taking a break from reading or doing any of the exercises is *always* an option. You can return to the material if and when you feel prepared again. Perhaps you will need to touch base with a therapist or a trusted friend before moving further. Before proceeding to chapter 1, please consider completing this opening exercise, which in the martial arts world we might call a *Prep Drill*. This exercise is here to be visited, built upon, added to, or subtracted from as you work through this book. While specific skills are taught for your use in the chapters that follow, we would feel most comfortable if you can jot down at least five items in this opening exercise before proceeding to chapter 1. Let this opening exercise be the safe enough harbor that you can return to at any time during your study.

Healing may seem difficult right now. Feeling this way is actually quite normal, whether you are new to the process of healing and recovery or have been at it for quite some time. We assure you, any journey can be much less intimidating if we take the time to prepare for it.

We thank you, from the bottom of our hearts, for including us in your process.

THE "SAFE ENOUGH" HARBOR AND OTHER GROUNDING EXERCISES

Recovery sponsors (mentors) will often say, "Write down a hundred things that make you feel good that do *not* involve drugs, alcohol, or acting out." Some examples include the freshness when you pop a mint into your mouth, or the potentially pleasant sensation when taking that first morning stretch. This exercise may require more than one sitting and can be visited and revisited over time. There is no pressure to come up with a hundred right now, so consider starting small—perhaps with five to ten items. Consider which of these activities can work for you as a refuge or a break if you need to take a pause while reading through this book or working on the exercises that will follow. Writing it down can make them more real, so please accept the invitation of this exercise as a necessary activity to keep yourself safe enough and supported through this work.

Keep a notebook, journal, or other loose paper nearby to make your list (and to keep adding to it). Having a journal dedicated to your work throughout *Dissociation Made Simple* can be a good idea for you in order to keep all of your activities organized. Such a journal is your private space and if there is not a safe enough space for you to keep it where you live, perhaps consider whether an alternative like the *Notes* feature on a password-protected phone might be viable. As a last resort, know that you have complete permission to safely burn or otherwise destroy any of the work that you do throughout this book if that feels safer for you. You will have gotten something out of writing it down, even if you then let it go.

One of the reasons that we use "safe enough" throughout the book is that we, and many other people struggling with complex trauma and dissociation, will literally roll our eyes if one more professional talks about a "Safe Place." Speaking for our system, the word *safety* is so loaded, and even in a state of recovery or wellness, safety is something we are always determining on a situation-by-situation and person-by-person basis. Also, because of the way the world operates, expecting someone to feel totally safe anywhere, even in their imagination, is unrealistic. So for us and for many we've worked with, thinking of skills, people, and resources as "safe enough" or "sufficiently safe" takes away the black-and-white of "I'm/we're either safe" or "I'm/we're not." Additionally, therapists may erroneously believe that a client has to feel totally safe or at least have a "Safe Place"–style resource to engage in deeper work. Again, such a construct may never be realistic. Speaking purely for ourselves, if we feel sufficiently safe with someone (e.g., a therapist, a person, a space), we can engage with them.

If you already know that you are working with a system, or different aspects of yourself, perhaps note which skills are best and most effective for certain parts of you. You may need to read chapters 4 and 5 first to obtain a better understanding of parts and systems, which is more than okay. You can always come back to this exercise after reading those chapters and add in additional skills for other parts that you may discover.

EXPRESSIVE ARTS PRACTICE: JAMIE'S SYSTEM AND PHOTOGRAPHY EXPLORATION

As we (Jamie) will describe throughout the book, there are many more parts and aspects of us that play out in our lived experience, yet the three major parts that are in the metaphorical car with me are *Four (Lucy)*, *Nine,* and *Nineteen.* We've expressed this metaphor in various expressive arts projects over the years (and we are blessed to have a trauma-focused therapist who practices many modalities, including art therapy). However, for the purposes of this book, since we are your guide, we thought it would be useful for you to see how we looked when we were chronologically four, nine, and nineteen. Because this is how Jamie sees and senses and feels their presence—along with all of their joys and sorrows and everything in between—as she navigates the car on this road of life.

As you learn more about your own system throughout this book or in your own therapeutic process, you may consider doing something similar with photographs. Trust your core judgment on whether this feels appropriate and safe enough for you at this time, remembering the grounding measures you have in place if the process of looking at photographs becomes too over-whelming or starts to cause an unhelpful shutdown in your system. You are in control of your healing process.

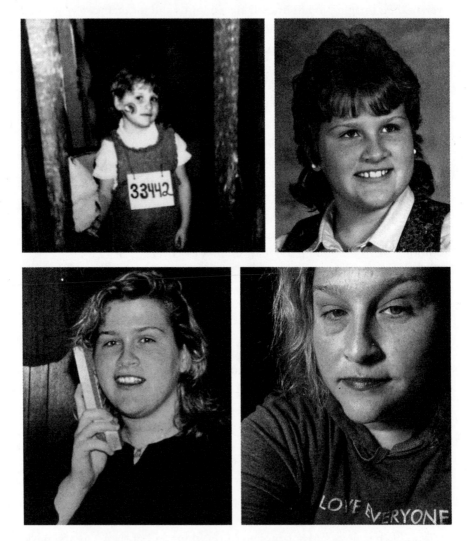

Top left (Four/Lucy); Top right (Nine); Bottom left (Nineteen); Bottom right (Jamie "The Driver," present day)

⸺QUESTIONS TO ASK MY THERAPIST OR PSYCHIATRIST⸺

- What is your approach to safety? Do you believe that it's an absolute construct (e.g., "I'm either safe or I'm not"), or do you believe safety is a more complex idea?
- What steps do you take in your practice to ensure that I am as safe as possible when engaging in the work?
- What is your working understanding of trauma and what approaches or techniques do you have in place for working with trauma?
- What is your general approach to working with dissociation?

HINT: If they say that they don't know what dissociation is or don't believe that it exists, we politely suggest that you seek out another provider, especially if the content of this book is already resonating with your lived experience. You may notice this ignorance around dissociation more frequently with psychiatrists, so finding one in your area who acknowledges dissociation may be difficult. At the very least, ask if they are willing to keep an open mind about how you describe your lived experiences and what you may be working on with your psychotherapist. You may also consider getting some tips from your therapist on how to advocate for yourself with the psychiatrist, or consider signing a release so that your therapist can communicate with your psychiatrist.

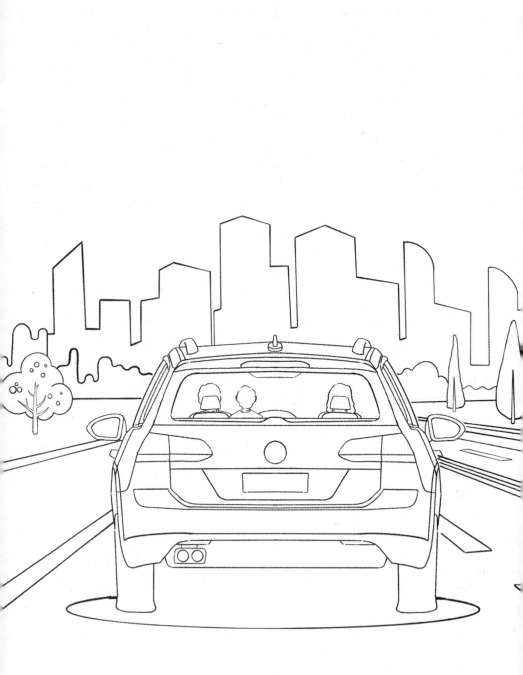

The Dance of Dissociation

To watch us dance is to hear our hearts speak.

—HOPI PROVERB

At this point in a book of this nature, the author is generally expected to lay out a series of definitions, peer-reviewed studies, neuroscientific theories, and rubrics from clinical manuals like the *Diagnostic and Statistical Manual of Mental Disorders* (DSM) or the treatment guidelines from the International Society for the Study of Trauma and Dissociation (ISSTD). Although I will do some of that here and in the chapter to follow, I find the task quite daunting. As a dancer, I know this feeling. There are so many steps that I could take, and my training tells me that I should choreograph them into some order that makes the most linear sense. Yet those kinds of dances really lack depth and soul. As we established in the introduction, so little about dissociation is linear. Others have tried, and by some counts succeeded in their studies and textbooks,* to explain it in an organized and linear fashion. As a very disso-ciative mind I find the task of codifying and classifying it nearly impossible.

---

* Please consult the Recommended Reading and Resources section at the end of this book for references to many of these works.

What makes it impossible is that dissociation is not just one thing. Continuing the dance metaphor, dissociation can be a series of steps, movements, and postures used in different combinations, and at different times. Sometimes those steps work gloriously, other times they do not, or they can even leave the dancer prone to injury if executed improperly, at the wrong time, or for too long a duration. The person who engages dissociation is the dancer; life is their partner. And life is an unpredictable and often cruel partner.

Pierre Janet understood this truth.

One of the criticisms lobbed against Pierre Janet, the French psychiatrist who formally coined the term *dissociation* in 1889, is that he did the best he could with what he had at the time, but tried to fit too much into one psychological construct. Some have conjectured, as summarized by James Fadiman and Jordan Gruber in their book *Your Symphony of Selves,* that the word Janet used in his native French, *désegrégation,* could have been better translated as "dis-aggregated." In English, an *aggregate* is a collection of parts into a whole, so the prefix *dis-* would suggest a breaking apart of that which has come together or is meant to stay together. However, the American philosopher William James would go on to translate it as "dissociation" in 1890, and by 1907 when Janet was lecturing at Harvard, he would continue to use this word.[1]

To be clear, there were documented cases of what we now call Dissociative Identity Disorder (DID) in clinical literature as far back as 1586, with the specific name "exchanged personality" later used in 1791.[2] The word *dissociation* was not created by Janet or those translating him; there is reference to Ahab's soul being "dissociated" from his mind in Herman Melville's 1851 novel *Moby-Dick.* However, Janet's use of it as a formal psychological phenomenon was revolutionary. According to trauma scholars Bessel van der Kolk and Onno van der Hart, Janet was the first to study dissociation as an organism's overwhelming response to trauma; specifically how unhealed trauma can manifest through wide-ranging and divergent sensory perceptions, affect states, and behavioral reenactments. Dr. Curt Rounazoin, a dissociation expert within the EMDR community and contributor to this book, explains candidly what makes Janet so important: "Janet believed his patients to his dying day, unlike Freud."

The explanation of Freud's movement toward theories of repression as an explanation for psychopathology or mental distress are well-known to those of us who work in mental health. Freud knew he was on politically shaky ground by validating the experiences of "hysterical" women who came to him discussing their premature sexual experiences. Many of these women were daughters of his elite colleagues at the University of Vienna, so he knew not to go there; and came to label what was really unhealed trauma as repression, "Oedipal complexes,"* and other defense mechanisms. The evidence apparent in Janet's writing and throughout his career really does position him as the father of trauma-focused approaches in modern psychology. Perhaps what made him most suited to this role is that he believed people and validated their lived experiences.

Defining Dissociation through Lived Experience

As a reader wanting to learn about dissociation, you are no doubt looking for more precise definitions. I will begin this section by presenting how we, as a dissociative system who is well-read on the scholarly technicalities of this topic, break down the definition and its intricacies to our students. And then, we will do what Janet did—listen to the people who were willing to come forward as contributors and speak of their lived experiences—to enliven the definitions and descriptions. Then we take a look at what some of the professionals who have powerfully validated our own lived experience offer in the way of a general definition.

Welcome to Jamie's Classroom: How We See It

To review from our introductory chapter, the English word *dissociation* comes from the Latin root *dissociātiō*, meaning "to sever" or "to separate." At this point when lecturing, I usually ask my students: What are we severing or separating from when we dissociate? You may take a moment, before reading on, to ask this question of yourself.

Try not to think on it too rationally.

Listen to your gut-level response.

In my own experience and in assisting others through my roles as a therapist and as a teacher, we are generally severing from one of two things in order to meet a need or to protect ourself/ourselves/our system. Yes, we may separate from our core self or develop more separate and distinct parts to help us deal with life. These experiences can be so intricate and

---

* A Freudian theory generally used to refer to a child's sexual desires for a parent of the opposite sex; largely rejected by empirical literature in modern times.

unique, I've dedicated an entire chapter (chapter 4) to further exploring this phenomenon and its manifestations. For the purposes of this opening chapter, let's focus on the form of separation that every human being can likely relate to—severing or separating from the present moment—especially when the present moment becomes unpleasant, overwhelming, or otherwise painful.

There are a variety of tasks that we either develop naturally or learn as a way to achieve some degree of separation (e.g., enough to stay somewhat present but still get some relief, or going further into totally cutting oneself off from in-the-moment presence). Dissociation of this nature is not all or nothing—it generally happens in degrees and can depend upon how much distress you feel in any given context. We can do this by daydreaming, drifting off, zoning out, zoning inward, disengaging eye contact with people, losing focus (especially when driving), or getting a little floaty in many other life circumstances. Some people frame this "floatiness" as similar to hypnotic trance and others feel it is quite distinct. We may even take deliberate steps to enhance the experience of separation. How often have you escaped into a book or a movie, into your phone or computer, or into some activity, because it makes the harshness of dealing with the present moment and the emotions it can elicit somewhat more bearable?

Let me be very clear, if you said yes to this question, this answer does not mean that there is anything wrong with you! All of these can be quite ordinary forms of dissociation that every human being is capable of experiencing. Using verbiage from the late Dr. Francine Shapiro, the creator of EMDR Therapy, these experiences can be *adaptive* (i.e., serving or helping us) or *maladaptive* (i.e., keeping us further stuck). She used these terms in describing responses to traumatic experiences (as opposed to terms like *healthy* or *unhealthy*) because she saw them as less of a value judgment and more honoring of an individual's subjective experience. In other words, what may be adaptive for you may not be adaptive for me; or what was adaptive at one time in my life might be different from what is adaptive now. And sometimes—the same behavior can still be both adaptive and maladaptive, depending on the context.

For you, having a glass of wine out on your porch after a hard day of work when you're feeling a bit crispy, or going out with your friends to do the same, may be a perfectly adaptive way to disconnect and to unwind. For me, as a person in long-term recovery from a substance use disorder who required abstinence to get well and to stay well, engaging in such a behavior can quickly lead to something maladaptive. Indeed for many of us, substances or other behaviors that cause major surges of dopamine (e.g., spending, computer games, sexually acting out) can become the accelerant of dissociation. In the 2000 film *28 Days,* Sandra Bullock's character Gwen Cummings writes, from rehab, to her boyfriend, asking him to bring her pills when he visits.

"That whole *here but not here* feeling will be much easier with a little bit of chemical assistance."[3]

That one line from a Hollywood movie succinctly captures what my colleague Adam O'Brien (also a trauma survivor and person in long-term recovery) has posited in our Addiction as Dissociation model.[4] Whenever we become accustomed to dissociating, especially as children growing up in complex trauma, our brain becomes bonded or some would even say *addicted* to that state of escape. Once chemical or other reinforcing behaviors are introduced to us, they can accelerate that already familiar experience and we become further bonded to that behavior. Speaking for myself, it's no wonder that once I reached eighteen months sober from alcohol and drugs, everyone around me started to notice significant dissociative symptoms. These symptoms fortunately led me to trauma treatment, where I was properly diagnosed.

I could make the case that drinking and drug use were very adaptive for me at one time because they kept me from actively ending my own life. Yet in the overall scheme of things, they were ultimately maladaptive because they kept me stuck in my trauma loops and caused their own sets of problems. Daydreaming and journeying into my head's imaginative scenarios is another series of behaviors that can have both adaptive and maladaptive qualities. As a kid, they kept me safe. As an adult, they are the source of so much of my creative power—yet if I engage them too long, too hard, or too much, I run the risk of getting lost and not being able to attend to what helping professionals might call my activities of daily living (e.g., eating properly, sleeping, taking good care of myself, getting to work, attending to loved ones appropriately and with good boundaries).

A final example I will offer you about dancing the line between adaptive and maladaptive dissociation is an insight into how I spend most evenings. After a hard day of work, I enjoy watching television or movies. Curled up on the couch with my cat Misty, engaging with these other worlds helps me to rest my body and actually feel some things—whether those feelings be elation and giddiness if I'm watching a comedy, or sadness and despair if I'm watching a drama. Even if my TV watching could be described as dissociative, for me it is not maladaptive because it is a refuge or separation that ultimately helps me to be more present for the rest of my life. I would argue that if I pushed through my evening and did more work or engaged in spiritual practices excessively to escape my feelings and my body's need to rest, that would be maladaptively dissociative.

The smartphone is another modern experience that can go both ways for people. Many of our contributors reported that having access to a smartphone as an instant dissociative coping device can help them in tense situations, like being at family gatherings or waiting in line at a crowded public place. Yet if the smartphone is keeping us chronically disconnected from aspects of life where we either need to engage or would be well-served to engage (e.g., fully experiencing a meaningful conversation with a friend or being attentive at work), then the dissociation might be more maladaptive or problematic.

Our Contributors' Perspectives

I am delighted that my personal therapist, Elizabeth Davis of Buffalo, New York, agreed to be interviewed as a contributor for this project; going on record with her name and sharing from her own life, too. I began working with Elizabeth in 2016 as my marriage was ending and I went through a self-injury relapse. Her knowledge of dissociation and refined training as an EMDR therapist and art therapist who intimately knows about the realities of spiritual abuse makes her the perfect fit for me. Elizabeth was brought up fiercely Pentecostal and poor in rural Appalachia, and maintains that finding visual art saved her.

"It was the only way to stay sane in my home," she shared.

Elizabeth's "clinical line" to define dissociation is that when our ability to stay present in life is disrupted, we default into states of denial or into other aspects of ourself/ourselves. Even though she recognizes that the clinical word *dissociation* is often incorrectly used by others when they pronounce it as "dis-association," she believes that the term *dis-association* is a relevant descriptor of what is happening. We are consciously or unconsciously cutting off association from some aspect of self or experience to manage or to cope. Sometimes we are dis-associating from vulnerability itself. Elizabeth believes that there is some aspect of dissociation in all clinical disorders. For her, dissociation showed up through Major Depression and an eating disorder in her twenties. Her eating disorder came from some need to dissociate from her body. Elizabeth reflects that even though dissociation was clearly present in both her eating disorder and Major Depression, the right questions were not asked at the time to help her frame it as such.

Another clinical professional interviewed for the project, John Fugett of the Pacific Northwest, also grew up in a fundamentalist Christian home that he sees as the source of his complex PTSD.

"Not the Christianity itself," he clarified, "But the *spare the rod, spoil the child* mentality."

John describes his therapeutic journey as being diagnosed with anything and everything *but* a dissociative disorder (an experience echoed by many other contributors). John even spent several years as a spokesperson and advocate for others with Bipolar Disorder, a diagnosis he carried for a long time that he now sees as unfounded. Once a new therapist began to explore dissociation with him, his healing came into a much greater sense of focus, and in fall 2020 he was diagnosed with Otherwise Specified Dissociative Disorder (OSDD).

While he says that how he explains his diagnosis continues to evolve, he attempts to make it as cognitive as possible for people: "Trauma and certain experiences cause neural networks to get split off, to the point that these networks don't have access to other individuals in the system. They don't get the advantage of having emotions modulated by other emotions in the system, and it can lead to a high degree of isolation."

John also describes depersonalization as a major component of how he experienced dissociation, noting, "When I am extremely depersonalized, I don't even know who John is. Dissociation, internally, allows me to feel separate, to watch the world from back here so that I can very quickly spot danger and get away from it."

Depersonalization is an expression of dissociation that can accompany DID or other dissociative disorders although it can also be classified as its own diagnosis (more in chapter 2). The same is true with the phenomenon called Derealization, a diagnosis that Andrea, another therapist contributor, can experience. In general, Andrea describes her relationship with dissociation as such: "I am so good at presenting fine in whatever situation I'm in. I'm good at being simultaneously fine and not fine. It takes me a long time to feel safe and show someone that I'm not okay."

For her, derealization makes her ask a great deal of questions about what is real and what is not real. A few months before our interview she said to her therapist, "I'm not sure if you're real," as she often sees the world in different situations from an outsider's perspective, something she's experienced since she was about six years old. She notes that this can make interpersonal relationships very difficult for her, as various parts in her system can make friends or engage in relationships that are not the healthiest for her overall. Yet a hope that she has held onto in her healing is that nature is real and animals are real. She literally goes to nature—to the earth, to the trees, to rivers—to get connected. For her and for many of us with dissociative disorders, it's people that can make things complicated.

For Jacqueline Lucas, the chronic pain that accompanies her fibromyalgia diagnosis complicates her life. In describing the interplay between her experience of complex trauma and fibromyalgia, "It's like being allergic to my own stress responses. With this comes brain fog, memory problems, and barriers to connection. It also makes it difficult to remember things and to formulate clear thoughts." Jacqueline describes dissociation as a double-edged sword: on one hand it is a useful tool that helps her cope, yet on the other hand it can make connecting with others very difficult.

Chuck Bernsohn, who also lives with a great deal of chronic pain, also finds that dissociation is a tool and a curse. Chuck describes, "I can totally disconnect from my body and do it with intention. But computer work can be dangerous for this reason, especially when I don't move for hours."

Working as an executive manager in addition to their work as an educator and advocate, Chuck often finds themselves at the computer!

Chuck, who simply defines dissociation as a spectrum, is a nonbinary individual who describes the intersection of their trans identity and their chronic pain as *dysphoria,* or a state of extreme dissatisfaction, anxiousness, and restlessness.

"My body doesn't always feel like my body," Chuck poignantly noted.

They went on to explain that the most gendered pieces of their body do not match up with how they see themselves in their head. This fundamental disconnect can be dissociative in and of itself, and can also be a factor in why individuals struggling to manage this disconnection may seek out, consciously or subconsciously, other ways to escape a very painful reality defined by separation. For many of our contributors, managing the confusion, the disorientation, and the disconnect becomes imperative. As you will discover throughout the book, my system has learned to do this in both adaptive and maladaptive ways, sometimes dancing between the two.

Many complex trauma survivors and those experiencing chronic illness or disabilities report a complicated relationship with the body that makes dissociation both vital and attractive. And for many of our contributors, like Destiny Aspen Mowadeng, when both complex trauma and illness or disability are present, dissociation is a literal lifeline. A certified trauma coach and disability rights advocate from Canada, Destiny was born with spina bifida. Due to her spinal cord injury and several other issues like hydrocephalus, Destiny has never been able to walk. She explains that because she's lived her life in a wheelchair, in situations where she cannot run physically, dissociation allows for some level of escape. Destiny, who survived a complex childhood in trauma and abuse at the hands of caregivers, simply defines dissociation as a disconnect that allows her to feel safe in the world; even if this means that she is sometimes looking at the world as if through a bubble.

Another advocate I had the pleasure of speaking to for this project is A.J., diagnosed formally with Otherwise Specified Dissociative Disorder (OSDD) and currently pursuing a graduate degree in clinical social work. A.J. is very well-studied on the intricacies of dissociation scholarship, and she identifies this project as being helpful in her own healing journey. About her background, A.J. says, "I am not my trauma but my trauma has informed almost everything about my adult life and there's no escaping that." When asked to describe dissociation, she has developed three layers of explanation, depending on the audience:

> To a kid I would say it's that feeling right after you wake up and you're not fully sure what's going on—kind of asleep and kind of awake. To a teenager I would say it's that space where you *zone out*. The difference between dissociating and normal zoning out is that there's a part of you that usually realizes you zoned out. With dissociation you can be left with this sense of—what happened? To the average adult I would stick with the adolescent metaphor but maybe introduce the language of autopilot even more. In its most dramatic form, dissociation is like being on autopilot but the ability to respond has been blunted.

From Our Trusted Colleagues

Being someone as outspoken as I am about many things, especially my own diagnoses and mental health struggles, navigating my professional circles can be a challenge. In the EMDR community many consider me a public figure because I have written three books specifically on EMDR, I have produced a great deal of video and media content, and I run one of the largest training programs currently on the market. Many EMDR clinicians look at me with a sense of awe about being so open, often saying things like, "Thank you for your vulnerability, Dr. Marich." Yet many other trainers and writers in the EMDR community have simply never addressed it with me, or are clearly uncomfortable when talking to me, especially about dissociation. Dissociative minds tend to embody a great deal of energetic sensitivity about whom we can trust and whom we cannot, and these signals ping strongly for us when interacting with others in our field. This theme of energetic sensitivity to how we experience others was also prominent in the interviews.

The four people from the EMDR community I asked to interview for this book project are not the only ones who have treated me with kindness and compassion about my coming out. Yet they are arguably the biggest names in terms of professional credibility who have most genuinely honored what we are doing to change the conversation about dissociation. And keeping it very real, our Four (Lucy) feels incredibly safe and seen when she is in their presence. We already introduced you to Dr. Curt Rounazoin, who acknowledges that the more intense the trauma, the greater the need to escape. In his interview he also disclosed a personal experience he had during a surgery around age eleven, where he was under anesthesia and shouldn't have been able to hear what the doctors were saying, but he clearly did. Says Curt, "That entire experience taught me that there is something more in our survival."

A second man from the EMDR community, a trainer who chose to remain anonymous in his interview, is a survivor of complex trauma. He sent us one of the most beautiful letters we ever received from a fellow professional and trainer, in response to our own disclosures made in print. In talking to him, I know that I am interacting with someone who understands dissociation from a very deep and personal place.

"A lot of my life is like I've been run through a tree chipper. I had really crazy people do really crazy things to me," he offered in plain and uncensored language.

He described dissociation as, *"An escape when there is no escape.* You do it not just to avoid pain and harm, it's what you need to do to survive."

Our entire system will never forget the genuine human kindness with which Dr. Debbie Korn, one of Dr. Francine Shapiro's early collaborators in EMDR Therapy, approached us after reading a very candid interview we gave to *Go With That* magazine about our personal lived experience.[5] Since then, we've been privileged to develop a friendship with Debbie and are impressed that, even though she does not identify as having a dissociative disorder or any major trauma history herself, she regards highly the inherent intelligence of dissociative clients and operates with a sense of fearlessness in treating us. Debbie defines dissociation as a universal phenomenon that is part of a response to overwhelming trauma that is essential to helping someone survive, maintain sanity, and continue to function. Dissociation is a protective response in the face of overwhelming and life-threatening (which can be subjective) circumstances.

Dr. Paul Miller, a psychiatrist from Northern Ireland trained during what is known as "the Troubles" in his native land, is one of the EMDR community's most progressive thinkers. The author of *EMDR Therapy for Schizophrenia and Other Psychoses,* he's published some innovative ideas about the interplay between psychosis and dissociation that we explore in chapter 2. On top of all of these achievements, Paul is a kind man with his own long history of evolving and growing as a person. Rich conversations about this growth process have formed the basis of our friendship. Moreover, I admire his ability to blend Western psychiatric training with a larger understanding of global consciousness and respect for non-Western methods of inquiry.

So when I asked Paul to define dissociation, he first offered a taxonomy of primary, secondary, and tertiary dissociation that he learned through his training and study with traditionally respected leaders in the field of dissociation studies, like Dr. Colin Ross. In primary dissociation there is no longer an integrated functioning of the brain. This phenomenon is something we all experience through behaviors such as daydreaming and lacking concentration, which we can do at times when we drive, while still fundamentally being safe. In secondary dissociation there is more of an out-of-body experience, a hard separation between participating and observing. This kind of dissociation has the potential to be more maladaptive or unsafe, yet it can be vital in getting people through crises. In tertiary dissociation there are clear and distinct parts at play and more of what's called a dorsal vagal response is activated. The dorsal vagal response, connected to the oldest nervous system in the human brain, can be described as a state where we are immobilized with fear, sometimes viewed as a hypoaroused state. In future chapters we further give voice to many of our contributors who believe that models and taxonomies like this are too boxed in, and that the polyvagal theory of Dr. Stephen Porges, which has popularized a term like *dorsal vagal state,* leaves much to be desired.

But Dr. Miller offered an even broader perspective that still gives us some semblance of organization, yet acknowledges that Western neuroscience does not hold all of the answers.

"There are unwell or sick people who hear voices. There are well people who don't hear voices. And there is a third—well people who hear voices. In Indigenous cultures, these are your healers and Shamans."

And indeed for many of us with intricate dissociative systems, the voices or felt senses that we experience come from within and can adaptively serve

our healing and promote genuine well-being and connection between ourselves and our world. Thus, in the next section we begin to explore the various other ways that dissociation shows up, adaptively and maladaptively, in
the dance that is the human experience.

Expanding Perspectives on Dissociation and Healing

All you have to do is look up *dissociation* in various online dictionaries and
you will see how it can mean different things in different contexts. Dictionary
.com, one of the online dictionaries that I consulted for this task, in defining dissociation as "separation," offered the following usage example: "the
dissociation of church and state."[6] As a spiritual abuse survivor who believes
ardently in this ideal, I nodded my head in agreement and declared, "Yes!
That is adaptive dissociation indeed! That's the kind of dissociation that we
need to *protect* people."

Yet in listening to our contributors, especially those with Indigenous ties
or who identify as people of color and/or not bound by the ties of Western
medicine, dissociation as it's been described so far in this chapter can mean
many things that are not helpful. A general consensus from these contributors is that trauma survivors ought never be shamed for doing what they
have to do in order to survive, especially because so many of the contexts into

Dissociation: In Their Own Words

Here are some other "one-liners" that additional contributors use to provide others with as succinct as possible a definition when asked: *What
is dissociation?*

"My brain becomes overwhelmed in certain situations or interactions;
it needs a break and I quickly go somewhere in space. Can feel like an
outside seizure."   —DANYALE WEEMS

"Most of the time it feels like a *time-out* on the inside of me. I need a
time-out and so I take it. I deal with my stuff but I need a time-out before I
can deal with it."   —SANDRA JOHNSON

which people are born promote division, disconnection, and marginalization. Usually this context is shaped by a dominant culture that relies on separation in its most unhelpful and wounding sense to uphold the power that the dominant culture so readily craves.

Let's turn to the voices of our contributors for even more nuance. As Wayne William Snellgrove sees it, *dis-association* begins in the environment of white colonialism. In his words, Wayne is a child of both roads, the Indigenous Red Road and the Western Colonial Road (having been adopted by white parents). A question he was left asking himself was, "How am I going to survive if I am a square peg and all I see are round holes?" For Wayne and for other Indigenous contributors to this book, there is no doubt that the historical and intergenerational trauma that all Native people experience left them exposed to developing addiction. And he is skeptical that the white colonial systems that promote separation, people staying asleep, power, and not living in harmony and balance can reliably help heal the damage they caused. He sees the Western model of healing as one of "fix me." Yet the Native or Indigenous path is one that requires you to get your hands dirty (literally by touching the earth), and teach one another how to reconnect in a beautiful way.

Jackson,* an African American veteran currently working as a therapist, grew up surrounded by a great deal of violence. He believes the problem of

---

* Pseudonym given to a participant who wishes to remain anonymous.

"The ability to separate, the ability to be outside myself; to hold those parts of myself. The parts of myself had to hold the pain to keep me alive." —SARAH SMITH

"Various degrees of feeling detached from myself and the world around me." —SUNNEE HOPE

"Dissociation is my body defending itself in certain situations." —ALEXIS

"An involuntary disconnect." —ERIN

"Dissociation is awesome! It's been helpful as an escape at times, but other times it's a problem." —CRYSTAL

violence among Black people is rooted in four-hundred–plus years of slave culture. He reflects, "You hurt people who look like you because the [dominant] system says that people who look like you don't matter." While he knows this phenomenon is not unique to Black communities, it is the "lane" of experience from which he is best able to speak. For Blaise Harris, an African American firefighter-turned-therapist who grew up in the American South, being taught to dissociate from his true feelings was what he needed to do in order to stay safe, especially from the threat of police violence. And if he was allowed to feel, happy or angry were the two choices. Once he began working in public safety, he noticed that more than half of his fellow firefighters were also disconnected or dissociated from their feelings in ways that were sadly more accepted by the dominant mainstream. Blaise offered, "We hide it with drinks, we hide it with work, we hide it with more work."

The sometimes controversial and always outspoken Japanese–Canadian somatics specialist and expressive artist Tada Hozumi offered various insights on how privilege, by its very definition, is dissociative. I sought him out a while ago as a consultant when I admired the way he called out how many Western practitioners miss the point about the true depth of embodied practices of marginalized peoples. Through his candor, I've learned so much about what really bothers me in our modern mental health systems and the ever broadening "wellness" industries. Even though many of us tout solutions for healing the impact of dissociation, are many of us still perpetuating the same

---

"Checking out is the first phrase that comes to mind. Separating yourself, not participating if you're somewhere you don't want to be."

—THE GARDEN SYSTEM

"An ability to be gone in different levels, different degrees, and in different ways."   —KATARINA LUNDGREN

"When my physical being is here but my mind is not in the present moment."   —REBECCA

"You're in this incredible trauma and you create this other sense of self to hold this for you so you can get on with your life."

—DIANNE HARPER

systemic garbage that creates the foundation for trauma to be perpetuated in the first place? And are those of us in the helping professions, especially those of us who are white and from dominant cultures, benefiting from the existence of a cultural dissociation?

Says Tada, "People who have all this level of technique but cannot tell their own story. That burns me up. And they never ask the elders in the traditions where so many of these techniques come from the questions that are important. That is cultural dissociation and disconnect." He also notes that circulation and ways of thinking that are nonlinear and non-hierarchical are frightening to a dissociated system. One of my dear friends and colleagues Susan Pease Banitt, a white female therapist steeped in the wisdom of her Celtic ancestry, made a similar offering: "Can you get a child at an early age and control their mind?" Intoning the wisdom of Alice Miller's *The Drama of the Gifted Child*, Susan notes that dominant cultures do this through early pedagogical control of the child's mind, that is based in shame and humiliation. It's no wonder that Susan describes herself as the kind of therapist who would rather hang out with Shamans than other therapists!

We will discuss some of the Shamanic and Indigenous perspectives on what often gets pathologized as "parts" or "alters" in chapter 4. For the purposes of this chapter it's most important to note how our contributors of color and even several white contributors who are responsibly connected to Native practices see the power-based culture's promotion of dissociation as a big part

---

"It's a trap door out of the present moment. It's an escape hatch for survival—for surviving what you don't feel like you can survive."

—DR. KELLIE KIRKSEY

"A way of trying to be okay in the world."   —ALICIA HANN

"I have an intellectual answer but my emotional answer is the inner compass; something that everyone is ignoring that could change the world. It helps me to find my truth."   —TANIYA

"To escape the prisoned moments or experiences."   —PAULA

"I am so disconnected that I can't connect."   —ANONYMOUS

of the problem in causing the kind of dissociation that does not serve us in the long run. Yet the same power structures can pathologize people who have defined "parts," using labels like DID, when so many of us are the carriers of wisdom and navigators between various realms of experience or even existence, at least as viewed through the lenses of these wisdom traditions. Julian Jaramillo, the Ecuadorian Shaman we met in the introduction, sees his job as one of building bridges between Indigenous paths of healing and Western psychology. And to help people rebuild bridges within themselves and to the communities that can facilitate their healing process. . . .

Roger Vielle, the Blackfeet elder we first met in the opening chapter, sees dissociation as just another word for confusion. This confusion can be promoted by society, especially by our political structures, or even marginalized people can do it to each other. He discussed how Native people will often use derogatory slurs with each other that question identity and commitment. The pain these slurs can cause creates dissociation, in Roger's view.

"Dissociation is caused by people dictating how they want to make you feel. There are times when people will naturally say *fuck it* and check out."

For Roger and many of our contributors, the solution to unhelpful dissociation is to promote a greater sense of *association*. Roger, a Vietnam-era veteran, has been leading other people—both Natives and non-Natives—in community-based healing practices like sweat lodge *(Inipi)* since he was himself incarcerated in the 1990s. As a man recovering from his own addiction, he believes that any way that we as people can get together without alcohol in a

---

"Walls that pop up around dimensions of our experience."
                                                            —CHRISTY DUNN

"A form of numbing out, separating one's self from what's going on; a self-preservation."   —MICHELLE KAHL

"When anything that my brain perceives as a threat or overwhelming becomes too much, a fogginess or severing from reality (well, half of reality) comes into my awareness."   —DANIELLE

spirit of reconnection and association is a significant part of the healing solution. More of these solutions for re-associating and promoting connection are fully explored in the chapters that follow, especially chapter 6.

Dissociation is a complicated word in our modern landscape because it can mean so many things, and there are many moving parts to navigate. As presented in the chapter opening, *the person who engages dissociation is the dancer; life is their partner. And life is an unpredictable and often cruel partner.* Carrying the metaphor a step further, the dance floor that is life and culture can make it very difficult to move in the most elegant way possible. There may be a lot of creaky and broken floorboards beneath us that people who can promote change never have a desire to fix. The systems in place that are ideally designed to help us dance might be creating more harm than good. Please remember that the next time you might judge yourself too harshly for your tendencies to dissociate. More importantly, remember this teaching if a person, especially one in a position of power over you or someone who would benefit from your collapse, tries to shame you for dissociating or for having defined parts.

We're all creating the dances that we can with the steps and conditions we've been given. If you've made it this far dancing as best as you can, my entire internal team truly salutes and honors you. We honor your struggle, and hope that you continue to get the insights that you need—either from this book or other sources you connect with along the way—to fully honor the beauty and fullness of what you've been able to create.

Survival is a creative process.

"At times it's for survival (conscious) and at times paralyzing (unconscious) . . . both leave me feeling hijacked."   —MALIKA

"Dissociation is like putting together a puzzle. You get a new puzzle, check to make sure it's safely sealed (so no contents are lost) then dump out the 1,000-plus pieces trying to organize them in such a way where you can create the full picture, so to speak. Slowly, and with some organized effort, it all comes together."   —BEEJAY

"It's our brain's way of giving us a break from stuff because of stress."

—OLGA TRUJILLO

EXPRESSIVE ARTS PRACTICE:
SURVIVAL IS A CREATIVE PROCESS

I realize that this chapter may have left you with more questions than answers, and that's part of my intention for writing the chapter in this way. In this closing expressive arts practice, you are invited to dance with, or otherwise engage with, some of what resonated for you in reading this content. We established that dissociation is a subjective construct (meaning different things to different people based on how we experience it). Sometimes dissociation is adaptive, sometimes it's maladaptive, and sometimes it can be both. Dissociation can be culturally sanctioned or enforced, and it can also help you survive or even navigate the impact of cultural trauma. And while you may be acknowledging that dissociation helped you to survive up until this point, you may also be regretting many of the ways that dissociation kept you cut off from life.

For this practice, we invite you to skim back over what you just read in this chapter, and write down three things that you related to the most. For those of you who naturally read with pencils, pens, and highlighters, you may have already done something similar. Using whatever expressive practice makes the most sense to you (e.g., dance/movement, listening to or making music, creative writing, visual art—which can include scribbling non-sensically), express what most resonates for you about these three concepts. Maybe, even if identified from several different places in the chapter, they are connecting in some way for you now.

HINT: If you're totally stuck, write down the three concepts on a separate piece of paper and literally dance around your space (with music or no music) with those concepts as your dance partner, and notice what's revealed.

After this expressive process draws to a natural conclusion for you, contemplate the phrase *survival is a creative act*. You can reflect on these questions in whatever way works best for you, although journaling (either with words alone or a combination of media) may help you further connect with the content:

- What can you appreciate about how any dissociative processes you may have engaged with up to this point in your life may have helped you to survive?

- What have these dissociative processes shown you about your strengths and your power, even if other people have tried to mock or shame you for engaging in such behaviors?
- How might the different frame you got on your behaviors and responses in this chapter, thanks to the wisdom of our contributors, help inform you for the path ahead?

QUESTIONS TO ASK MY THERAPIST OR PSYCHIATRIST

- What is your working definition of *dissociation?*
- What connection do you see between dissociation and survival?
- Even though you work in these helping professions, do you recognize where certain aspects of your profession may be doing more harm than good? Or directly promoting unhelpful dissociation?
- Are you willing to help me discover my own working definition of *dissociation* as we go forward together in our work?
- What have your own clients taught you thus far about the reality of dissociation and how to work with its impact?

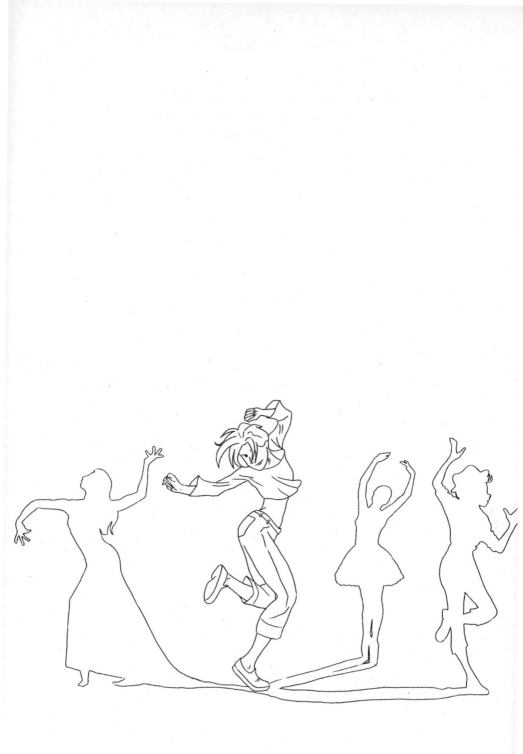

2

So, Is There Anything Really Wrong with My Brain?

Our minds, due to their nature as a spark or wave of a much greater, infinite intelligence, are capable of unbelievable things.
—CHRISTINA SARICH

I found this chapter the most difficult in the entire book to write. As I voiced in the introduction, when I consult clinical and scientific literature on dissociative disorders and neuroscience, it feels like I am being turned into a science project. Who I am/we are as a person is so much more than the physical body. And what compounds this difficulty is that so many factions of the behavioral health professions and in society at large want this hard science, complete with brain imaging scans and empirical data, to prove the very existence of a mind and a way of being in the world that has always been very real to me. Even when I consult literature by leading scholars like Dr. Bethany Brand and Dr. Milissa Kaufman, champion researchers for people with dissociative disorders whose work many contributors to the book consider important and significant, I feel like I'm reading the transcript of a fight over the validity of trauma and its impact on human beings. Brand, a psychologist who can make a case as skillfully as any lawyer, and Kaufman, a psychiatrist with both an

MD and a PhD, use empirical evidence, the latest neurological technology, and peer-reviewed studies to support the existence of trauma-related dissociation and the utility of diagnosing and treating its manifestations. They need this depth of evidence to inevitably counter claims by others who also attempt to use empirical evidence and studies to argue differently.

Peer-reviewed (a term meaning that other scholars have approved a paper for publication in an academic journal) and *evidence-based* (a term meaning that an approach or series of treatments has sufficient peer-reviewed data to receive backing from a clinical organization) are important concepts in the modern behavioral health professions. Yet they fundamentally represent a binary way of thinking as defined by the dominant culture. In a controversial social media and website post that was later taken down, the National Museum of African American History and Culture identified the rational, linear thinking and quantitative nature of research based only in the scientific method as a fundamental aspect and assumption of white culture in the United States.[1] Dr. Sand Chang, a nonbinary mental health practitioner and growing social media influencer, gives a direct explanation of what makes this a problem:

> There is no single "right" way to do therapy or healing work—assuming "evidence-based practice" is superior to all other approaches (including Indigenous practices) is dehumanizing. Keep in mind that many approaches that have been presented as "evidence-based" or based on "objectivity" have contributed to the harm or genocide of BIPOC, trans people, disabled people, neurodivergent people, fat people, and other marginalized groups.[2]

And there are more reasons a solely scientific approach to understanding the human mind is insufficient. An Infinite Mind,* the premier advocacy organization founded for people with DID and dissociative disorders by Jaime Pollack, a preschool teacher with DID who contributed the foreword to this book, puts it right out there on their website: The brain is merely an organ, but the mind is infinite.[3]

In my own work as a mindfulness educator over the years, I've entertained the debate between what is the brain and what is the mind, a debate that goes all the way back to Aristotle and Plato. Yogic philosophy clearly describes mind as activity, or vibrating energy, not a physical entity like the brain. Descartes called the brain the seat of intelligence, which can distinguish itself from the mind, which holds a consciousness and self-awareness of itself.

---

* Go to www.aninfinitemind.com for more information.

Christina Sarich, the journalist and yoga scholar whose quotation opens this chapter, describes the mind as capable of creating substance from nothingness. She writes:

> It contains the aura, or energy body, and can project to other minds, and receive from them also. It communicates in the language of feeling. It has a profound effect on the energy level of the physical body, which temporarily houses it, and has the capacity to heal its own physical house as well as that of others.[4]

As I wrote in my 2015 book *Dancing Mindfulness: A Creative Path to Healing and Transformation,* in an attempt to navigate the debate myself: "The brain is the biological instrument that houses the mind and allows for its function. However, to describe 'the mind' is so much more multifaceted and wondrous than just rendering it synonymous with the brain."[5]

I've long stood by my teaching on brain versus mind, and a theme expressed through many contributors to the book is that there is so much more going on in the spiritual or energetic realm for people with dissociative disorders, as labeled by Western psychology. Dr. Curt Rounazoin, a recognized expert on dissociation whom we've met in previous chapters, articulates that there is an aspect of dissociation that is beyond the brain. He says, "There is a spirit of light and life and something took it away. You don't have to be religious to be open to the fact that trauma is a spiritual issue." For Jasa Johnson, a Shamanic practitioner who guides people through healing journeys like soul retrieval on a regular basis, people can be hesitant to look at the spiritual aspects of what ails them because spiritual practice (not to be confused with religion) is not valued by dominant cultures. There can be an attachment to believing only in what you can see around you, or on a brain scan, as real. She continues, "People are frightened that they are not worthy of goodness or blessings. If they want to stay stuck in the science, I'm happy to leave them there."

For Destiny Aspen Mowadeng, the advocate and trauma coach living in a wheelchair due to her congenital spina bifida: "I'm science's fucked up failure. I'm the thing they tried to fix and couldn't." Several years back I gave an interview on a podcast about dissociation and in a flow of inspiration I said, "We've pushed the science so hard, the soul has been missing." The very next day, Destiny made a meme of this teaching and shared it on social media; it remains one of her favorite ideas in my work. For Destiny, who is angered by phrases we use in the trauma recovery field like *the body keeps the score* (based on the title of Bessel van der Kolk's 2014 book), trauma is more than the physical body and more than science. Destiny and several other contributors say that any suggestions that trauma is only about the body or only about the brain reeks of eugenics, or the idea that people with disabilities or "defects" automatically need to be improved or fixed, especially so that more defects are not created in ongoing populations. The suggestion of van der Kolk's title that human processes are some kind of game is resented by many who spoke with me, even though many others who contributed highly value the book and its concepts.

And this is where Dr. Jamie has engaged in quite the debate with Jamie throughout the preparation and writing process for this book. Jamie wants to *go there* about the spiritual and even metaphysical aspects of trauma and dissociation because after all, it's Jamie who gets disgusted by what she hears at academic conferences and reads in journals. It's Jamie who believes that what gets presented in the clinical mainstream is only telling part of the story. And then Dr. Jamie expresses her concern, afraid that the field won't take this book seriously enough if there is too much emphasis on the spiritual and mystical elements of dissociation and not enough emphasis on the *brain science*. She is also concerned that some of you picking up this book might need the science to be convinced that your symptoms are valid and that you are worthy and deserving of the help that you seek. Especially if part of your abuse was religious or spiritual in nature, and encountering anything beyond hard science and factual evidence can be triggering. . . .

Talk about dissociation!

So in keeping with the overall style of this book, we are choosing to lean into the voices of our contributors to help navigate the necessary sections of this chapter—examining topics like trauma, dissociation, the brain, and clinical diagnoses. This chapter is our attempt to present this very relevant information with the soul that has been lacking. We will certainly give you information— because there is plenty of it available—on where you can learn more about trauma, dissociation and the brain, clinical diagnoses, and the latest scholarship in the field. We elected to keep the focus more on what our contributors and their lived experiences had to say in illuminating this content than rehashing what is already out there. So please be sure to visit the Recommended Reading and Resources section for much more information on everything covered in this chapter, most of which can be freely obtained online.

What's Happening in My Brain?

As we begin our conversation around the neuroscience of dissociative processes, it would seem prudent to start with some of the basic neuroscience of trauma. Yes, unhealed human wounding can change the brain if the wound is not given a chance to process or heal at the time it experienced the wound. And the systems and parts of the brain that are most involved in helping our bodies navigate trauma and its aftereffects have little to do with words and rational thought. The two predominant models that many modern trauma scholars lean into for explaining the neurobiology of trauma are the triune brain model or hand model of the brain, based on the work of Dr. Paul McLean and later popularized by Dr. Dan Siegel; and poly-vagal theory, the work of Dr. Stephen Porges. While both models are still in use (and I have used them throughout my work), there is ample criticism in the literature about each lacking nuance and detail, and several of our contributors express that they feel both models paint an incomplete picture about dissociation.

We start with the basics of each model simply to assemble some vocab-ulary. Then, we will turn to my EMDR Therapy colleague, psychiatrist Dr. Paul Miller, for how he sees this all coming together with the recognition that many systems are at play in attempting to understand dissociation at the level of the brain. Dr. Miller also recognizes that helping professionals, psychia-trists especially, can feel very insecure about trying to explain the power of the human mind and the *art* of therapy. This insecurity can create a tendency for us to explain exactly what is going on within the anatomical brain to justify how we work. Yet as Dr. Miller cautions, citing the wisdom of his friend (and neuroscientist) Dr. Uri Bergmann, the focus has got to be on how everything works together. For us to properly engage in this discussion, it is relevant at this point to also discuss how dissociation shows up in other clinical diagno-ses besides the dissociative disorders, and how everything can interplay.

Let's start with the "three brains" that constitute the triune brain:

- The brain stem (sometimes called the reptilian brain, although brain stem is more correct): includes the cerebellum (the struc-ture at the bottom of the brain that plays an active role in motor control and sensorimotor processes); controls instinctual survival behaviors, muscle control, balance, breathing, and heartbeat. Very reactive to direct stimuli, and most associated with the freeze to submission response and other hypoarousal and dissociative experiences like collapse, and what is sometimes called fawn-ing. Fawning can be described as giving in and doing whatever another wants just to keep the peace, or to achieve some perceived experience of attachment or affection.

- The limbic brain (sometimes called the mammalian brain, the learning brain, or the heart brain): contains the amygdala, hypothalamus, hippocampus, and the nucleus accumbens (responsible for dopamine release). The limbic system is the source of emotions and instincts within the brain, responsible for fight-or-flight responses. Emotion is activated by input in this brain. Everything in the limbic system is either agreeable (pleasure) or disagreeable (pain). Survival is based on the avoidance of pain and the recurrence of pleasure.

- The neocortex (or cerebral cortex): is unique to primates and some other highly evolved species like dolphins and orcas. This newest region of the brain regulates our executive functioning—which can include higher-order thinking skills, reason, speech, and sapience (i.e., wisdom, calling upon experience). The limbic system needs to interact with the neocortex in order to process emotions. When the limbic system is overactivated (hyperarousal) or the brain stem creates a sense of shutdown, or collapse (hypoarousal), this process can prove difficult because blood flow suspends in some way to the left prefrontal cortex (responsible for making sense of things and processing information) even though the right brain (responsible for awareness) can remain online. A healthy brain relies on integration between left and right brain hemispheric activity, and dissociative responses activated at the brain stem can disrupt this balance.

Polyvagal theory now informs how many trauma therapists assist their clients to more effectively heal their nervous systems. Porges explains, "Mammals . . . evolved in a hostile environment in which survival was dependent on their ability to down regulate states of defense with states of safety and trust, states that supported cooperative behavior and health."[6] The vagus nerve—the long nerve canal that extends from the brain, down the spine, linking the brain to our vital organs—is essential to understanding polyvagal theory and the brain–body link in trauma work. *Vagus* comes from the Latin word meaning "to wander" or "to travel."

Clinical social worker Deb Dana[7] breaks down the three main components of polyvagal theory: autonomic hierarchy, neuroception, and co-regulation. Autonomic hierarchy is the organization of the nervous system from oldest to newest. The dorsal, or rear side, of the vagus nerve formed 500 million years ago in the earliest animals and is responsible for mobilization strategies and part of the parasympathetic nervous system. Next, 400 million years ago, came the sympathetic nervous system, which is responsible for fight and flight. The ventral (or front) side of the vagus nerve, formed 200 million years ago. Also part of the parasympathetic nervous system, the ventral vagal state is responsible for social engagement. Dana explains that when our ventral vagal state is activated, our body–mind complex is most receptive to healing and change. *Typically when we are dissociated, we are in a dorsal vagal state.*

Neuroception suggests that the body can work below the level of awareness to give us information at an implicit level. Jamie has long told her clients, "Your body will alert you to what's going on ten steps before you even realize that anything is the matter." This teaching exemplifies neuroception. In keeping with the theme of this chapter, more than just the physical body might be at play. Your energetic sensibilities, or what we sometimes call *vibe*, spirit, or anything paranormal (beyond the normal) can be factors.

Co-regulation teaches that all mammals are in the best position to stay regulated and balanced when they have consistently engaged in this behavior with others. We, as people and as mammals, attune to each other's nervous systems. This is the reason why you can have a very meaningful relationship with your pet—without ever having to exchange any words. A major reason that trauma therapists speak to the power of the calming presence is that such a presence can be a healing intervention in and of itself, explained by co-regulation. In the chapters that focus on treatment, many of the people we spoke to for this book share how important this presence on the part of their therapist is for them in the healing process.

Dr. Paul Miller cautions us not to reduce understanding dissociation and the brain down to one area or one phenomenon being investigated. Doing a full literature review on everything being looked at right now around the neuroscience of dissociation would exceed the space that I have available in this book, and would defeat the purpose of the more artistic approach that I'm taking with the material. While this abundance of research* is part of what can add to my frustration, I find that Dr. Miller's teaching that there are a variety of factors involved gives me some peace. All of these show that I and others like me are not just "making this up." He noted that first the focus of the research seemed to be on the amygdala, and then it focused more on memory and the role of the

---

* Be sure to visit the Recommended Reading and Resources section for full recommendations on where you can track the latest research.

hippocampus. Citing the triune brain model, Dr. Miller also notes that dissocia-tive responses, which can originate in the brain stem as a more primal response, inhibit right–left hemispheric communication. He notes, "This creates a prob-lem with the embodied sense of being in the world. And then you end up with this very left-hemisphere–dominant presentation, where things are reduced down to an assemblage of parts. Literally a definition of dissociation."

Dr. Miller is also well-known for his work of conceptualizing schizophrenia and other psychotic disorders through the lens of dissociation. His book *EMDR for Schizophrenia and Other Psychoses* is a master class in looking at the history of diagnosis within the psychiatric professions in a more dissociation-informed way. When asked to differentiate the difference between psychosis and dissoci-ation, he bluntly answered, "They're the same thing."

The psychotic disorders like schizophrenia and schizoaffective disorders are typically identified by their reality testing in the form of delusions or hallu-cinations. *Psychosis*, which comes from the Greek root meaning "animation of life," is generally seen to be more organic in nature, meaning there is a defect or issue in the brain that is not directly related to trauma or stress. People with psychotic disorders may not be amenable to the insights of psychotherapy, although general psychosocial support tends to be most helpful. Yet over the years Miller has treated a variety of patients with trauma histories (who tech-nically carry psychotic diagnoses) that are very responsive to trauma-focused psychotherapies either in addition to or in place of their medication manage-ment. And thus begins our look into the question of whether dissociation is present in all forms of psychiatric diagosis. And when dissociative disorders or presentations are there in addition to other disorders, what does this all mean for trying to make sense of what's happening in the brain?

Cheryl is one of our contributors who identifies as having been diagnosed with both schizoaffective disorder (a psychotic disorder) and DID. Cheryl is a factory worker from Canada. Her therapist, who she describes as having saved her life for properly diagnosing and treating the DID, primarily works with her on that diagnosis. Her psychiatrist sees her as having a schizoaffec-tive diagnosis with dissociation, and she does find the lithium and Invega that she is prescribed to be helpful, especially in eliminating the presence of what she describes as "spies" and helping her get a better quality of sleep. Yet the treatment that's focused on the DID has helped her to make sense of symp-toms like losing time and being on what she describes as autopilot. For her, all of the symptoms in both diagnoses are trauma-related and she benefits greatly from an integrated treatment approach.

Just as Dr. Miller said very definitively that psychosis and dissociation are one and the same (although there may be variations in how they manifest), contributor Adam O'Brien and I would answer as definitively about addiction and dissociation—that they are one and the same. This contention is the basis for our Addiction as Dissociation model, first published in 2019.[8] One of the reasons we saw the need for this model is to promote a better, more trauma- and dissociation-informed presentation of the word *addiction*. The word *addiction* has come under criticism in the modern era because many feel that term is stigmatizing and not adequately trauma-informed.[9] In response, the Addiction as Dissociation model offers this definition of *addiction:* "the relationship created between unresolved trauma and the continued and unchecked progression of dissociative responses." In presentations where primary addiction treatment has failed to address trauma, dissociative experiences will inevitably produce a dissociative disorder or clinically significant symptoms of dissociation. Similarly, if "dissociation in trauma"[10] has not been treated accordingly, addiction will inevitably manifest. The model contends that addiction can only develop in relation to trauma and dissociation because trauma (cause) produces dissociation (effect).

According to the *dissociation in trauma* concept of Ellert R.S. Nijenhuis and Onno van der Hart, there is a "division of an individual's personality, that is, of the dynamic, bio-psychosocial system as a whole that determines his or her characteristic mental and behavioral actions."[11] This distinction can also be seen in the Waller, Putnam, and Carlson analysis regarding nonpathological and pathological (i.e., adaptive and maladaptive) dissociative traits, of which dissociation in trauma would be represented by the latter.[12] *In plain language, dissociation is what creates safety and ultimately pain relief in the moment of need. Trauma deeply impacts a person's psyche, extreme limits are pushed, and extreme reactions become necessary.*

Mergler, Driessen, and Ludecke and colleagues examined the relationship between the PTSD Dissociation subtype (new to the DSM-5) and other clinical presentations. In a sample of 459 participants, the dissociative subtype group demonstrated a statistically significantly higher need for treatment due to drug problems, in addition to higher current use of opiates/analgesics, and a higher number of lifetime drug overdoses. They ultimately concluded that dissociative subtype is related to "a more severe course of substance-related problems in patients with substance use disorders, indicating that this group also has additional treatment needs."[13]

Dr. Miller, in his explanation of various brain processes involved with dissociation, names several researchers that people interested in the neurobiology of DID ought to check out, like Simone Reinders and Yolanda Schlumpf. He points to the work of Drs. Ulrich and Ruth Lanius and their research (along with various colleagues) around the endogenous opioid system. In various forms of functional brain scans, the areas that show up as most active in terms of dissociation are rich in endogenous opioid receptors (found in the limbic system). You can think of our endogenous opioid system as our body's natural defenses it can muster against pain, yet people often find that taking euphoria-producing medications or drugs can amplify the potency of this system. The endogenous opioid system can produce internal trauma reenactments as external stressors trigger the internal neurochemical processes that produce unconscious behaviors like dissociation and addictive processes (i.e., kill the pain now).[14] Further demonstrating how intricately linked these processes are, the medication naltrexone (at low dosages) has shown to be helpful in treating both dissociative disorders (whether or not the patient has an addiction issue) and the treatment of alcohol and opioid dependence because naltrexone blocks opiate receptors.[15]

There are two contributors who came forward to be interviewed for the book specifically because they resonated with the Addiction as Dissociation model. Megan is a thirty-three-year-old Caucasian woman from the American South who works in the field of emergency medical services; she identifies a DID diagnosis and a history of being treated for substance use disorder. At the time of her interview for this book she identifies several years of sobriety from alcohol. For Megan, while working in emergency medical services (a career to which she has recently returned in an administrative capacity), dissociation wasn't something she could "do," but drinking became something that brought her relief and was seen as more acceptable on her days off. Megan originally thought her work was the sole source of her PTSD, but the more she began exploring that in trauma-focused treatment, the layers revealed themselves and a diagnosis of DID started to make more sense.

Megan describes her DID as, "I have parts. I have a group of people inside of me that present as the person that you see. But internally it's a completely different person. These parts were created from childhood trauma and their purpose was to protect me. They work together (mostly) to continue to protect me."

Kylie, a newer therapist who is a survivor of childhood religious and sexual trauma, does not carry a DID diagnosis but dissociation resonates for her because of her past struggles with alcohol. She defines dissociation as "a falling asleep to yourself, abandoning yourself; leaving the present that is too much." In her words, the addiction as dissociation connection played out as such: "the drinking was a way not to feel or think about the deep emotional pain that I was feeling; it was a way to feel better, to ease the pain." Rebecca, a contributor who is a survivor of complex childhood trauma, still reports long-term concussion syndrome resulting from her childhood abuse. For Rebecca, a woman who reports five years of sobriety from alcoholism and narcotic addiction (which largely developed in response to medical issues), connecting the dots of addiction as dissociation was an "aha" moment.

Rebecca never felt a previous connection with the 12-step concept of "I'm an alcoholic" or "I'm an addict," and long believed, inherently, that her addiction issues were a response to childhood trauma.

For my professional collaborator and contributor to this project Adam O'Brien, in describing his personal experiences with dissociation, addiction, and what is happening in the body–mind complex, he comments:

> Originally what it feels like is an out-of-body experience but there is a gradual lifting off where there is a level of co-consciousness where you can experience *and* witness it. In the brain it's a numb state, but also safe ... when I first took a drug, it reminded me of the safety I first had during my near-death experience at age four ... without judgment or recourse, it just *was* ... being in an all-knowing space. Not bliss, but could be similar to the feeling of "getting high," injecting inward into the body.

For Adam, the word *dissociation* doesn't quite capture what is happening. He continues, "My current thinking is God—it's where you go when things here aren't okay, and it takes care of you."

How Dissociation Shows Up in a Variety of Diagnoses

In various cultures, certainly in Indigenous paths of inquiry, Adam's description makes complete and total sense. For Julian Jaramillo, the Shaman we met in previous chapters, diagnosis can be beautiful in their system because it seeks to embrace a person's mythology for understanding why, in his words, a person's "head is hurting." In the system of Western psychology and psychiatry, diagnosis has long sought to codify how groups of signs and symptoms together might be causing impairment in an individual's life so that the best course of treatment can be prescribed. Contributors to the book have mixed feelings about diagnosis. On one hand there is a belief that "who I am as a person or as a system is more than just my diagnosis," and many of these feelings are presented in chapter 7, on removing stigma. While the Western diagnostic system can certainly be criticized for labeling and pathologizing people, for many of our contributors getting a correct diagnosis or series of diagnoses that took trauma and dissociation into account was empowering, validating, and helped them accept the most meaningful treatment possible. In this section we will take a look at the specific diagnoses that fall into the American Psychiatric Association's *Diagnostic and Statistical Manual of Mental Disorders* (DSM-5) chapter on dissociative disorders specifically. Then we will continue our exploration of how dissociation may show up in other diagnoses with various intersections (e.g., between dissociation and neurodivergence) also being discussed.

The Dissociative Disorders

For an individual to meet any of the diagnostic criteria that follow, the dissociation must not be better explained by a phenomenon like intoxication, or what certain cultures may call possession. You can consult a copy of the DSM-5 to read the specific diagnostic criteria that cannot easily be reprinted here due to copyright restrictions. We provide ideas on where to find this information in the Recommended Reading and Resources section. I am able to offer you these very solid summaries of each diagnosis involved as presented by An Infinite Mind (used with permission).* Please be sure to consult the inset for how some of our contributors describe their diagnosis in their own words.

- Dissociative Identity Disorder (DID)

    DID, formerly called multiple personality disorder, develops as a childhood coping mechanism. To escape pain and trauma in childhood, the mind splits off feelings, personality traits, characteristics, and memories into separate compartments that then develop into unique personality states. Each identity can have its own name and personal history. These personality states recurrently take control of the individual's behavior, accompanied by an inability to recall important personal information that is too extensive to be explained by ordinary forgetfulness. DID is a spectrum disorder with varying degrees of severity. In some cases, certain parts of a person's personalities are aware of important personal information, whereas other

---

* For more, see www.aninfinitemind.com/about_DID.html.

personalities are unaware. Some personalities appear to know and interact with one another in an elaborate inner world. In other cases, a person with DID may be completely aware of all the parts of their internal system. Because the personalities often interact with each other, people with DID report hearing inner dialogue, and the voices will comment on their behavior or talk directly to them. It is important to note the voices are heard on the inside versus the outside, as this is one of the main distinguishers from schizophrenia. People with DID will often lose track of time and have amnesia around life events. They may not be able to recall things they have done or account for changes in their behavior. Some may lose track of hours while some lose track of days. They have feelings of detachment from themselves and feelings that their surroundings are unreal. While most people cannot recall much about the first three to five years of life, people with Dissociative Identity Disorder may have considerable amnesia for the period between the ages of six and eleven as well. Oftentimes, people with DID will refer to themselves in the plural (e.g., "we").

- Dissociative Amnesia

  The most common of all dissociative disorders and usually seen in conjunction with other mental illness, dissociative amnesia occurs when a person blocks out information, usually associated with a stressful or traumatic event, leaving them unable to remember important personal information. The degree of memory loss goes beyond normal forgetfulness and includes gaps in memory for long periods of time or loss of memories involving the traumatic event.

- Depersonalization Disorder

  Having depersonalization has sometimes been described as being numb or in a dream, or feeling as if you are watching yourself from outside your body. There is a sense of being disconnected or detached from one's body. This often occurs after a person experiences life-threatening danger, such as an accident, assault, or serious illness or injury. Symptoms may be temporary or persist or recur for many years. People with the disorder often have a great deal of difficulty describing their symptoms and may fear or believe that they are going crazy.

- Unspecified Dissociative Disorder (UDD)

  Symptoms do not meet the full criteria for any other dissociative disorder, and the clinician chooses not to specify the reason that the criteria are not met.

- Otherwise Specified Dissociative Disorder (OSDD)

  The Otherwise Specified Dissociative Disorder category is used in situations in which the clinician chooses to communicate the specific reason that the presentation does not meet the criteria for any specific dissociative disorder.

  OSDD is sometimes referred to as a "catch-all" diagnosis (similar to the former Dissociative Disorder, Not Otherwise Specified in the previous edition of the DSM) for clusters of symptoms that do not neatly fit any of the other diagnoses. The DSM-5 identifies four subtypes of OSDD, summarized in my words as:

  - Type 1: Closest to DID yet not meeting full diagnostic criteria for DID; another diagnostic system, the International Classification of Diseases (ICD-11th revision) refers to this as "partial dissociative identity disorder." Some scholars take this a step further, distinguishing OSDD-1a (separate and distinct parts but with not enough separation to qualify as what's been

---

In Their Own Words: DID

"DID has been a practice to maintain awareness. Even when we're fluid with who is present. It's not like *Split* though; there is no serial killer going to come and hack off your face. It is like having a body bus. I'm driving the bus. I can step away from the wheel and one of them takes over."

—HEATHER (LS) SCARBORO+ *(diagnosed with DID)*

"It feels like the DID, especially earlier on in therapy, that my brain was broken up into compartments and I could pinpoint where everybody lived, everybody had their own little compartments. Now that I've had so much therapy there is a difference; there are tiny little boxes with no all-access pass."   —JAIME POLLACK *(diagnosed with DID)*

traditionally called alters) and OSDD-1b (no amnesia between parts with switching rarely or never happening).[16]

- Type 2: Distressing changes to or questioning of their identity, usually due to long-term brainwashing or coercion (e.g., cults, political imprisonment, thought reform programs).

- Type 3: Constriction of consciousness, which can last from a few weeks up to a month; can include depersonalization, derealization, perceptual disturbances, time slowing, objects appearing closer and larger than they really are, micro-amnesia, alterations in sensorimotor functioning.

- Type 4: Dissociative trance or, according to the DSM-5, acute narrowing or complete loss of awareness; profound unresponsiveness. This presentation is valid if it's not better explained by religious or cultural practices.

For many of us with dissociative disorders, especially OSDD, it can feel like different criteria may apply at different times in our lives. And many of us have developed an interesting system of metaphors to explain what the internal system feels like, most of these being explored more fully in chapter 5. Contributor Susan Pease Banitt, who shares from both personal and professional experience, offers this useful metaphor to help us make a distinction:

"DID is the brain's ultimate defense mechanism that I used when I was young. I have different parts of my brain that are sectioned off. I don't do what people see on TV or in the movies—like switching in the middle of the day or changing my clothes."

—ALEXIS *(diagnosed with DID)*

"A big family in your head you have to get along with. And we are getting along better than we used to."

—THE GARDEN SYSTEM *(diagnosed with DID)*

"The brain is a huge network—it's a different hub for different things. Sometimes communication is cut off between hubs."

—KATARINA LUNDGREN *(diagnosed with DID)*

"Imagine a big room with a cubicle with it; in a 'normal' brain there are cubicles like in an office, but with forms of DID the walls are so high they are soundproof. With OSDD the walls go most of the way to the ceiling but not all the way."

Complex PTSD and Other Diagnoses

The *Diagnostic and Statistical Manual* (DSM) is used by clinical professionals to guide diagnosis. In the fifth edition (2013), a new chapter of Trauma- and Stressor-Related Disorders (which includes PTSD, acute stress disorder, adjustment disorders, reactive attachment disorder, and disinhibited social engagement) does make mention of dissociative symptomology as a potential feature of PTSD. In the DSM-5 version of the PTSD diagnosis, there is a qualifier option: PTSD with Predominant Dissociative Symptoms. Dissociation can play out in all five symptom areas of the PTSD diagnosis, with flashbacks (under Criterion B, reexperiencing) specifically being described as a dissociative phenomenon. The other symptom areas include avoidance of stimuli associated with the trauma (Criterion C); alterations to cognition and mood (Criterion D); and hyperarousal symptoms like a heightened startle response, problems paying attention, or sleeping (Criterion E). Criterion A is the qualifying trauma itself—a life- or injury-threatening event, sexual violation, or other experience that can include witnessing a traumatic event happen to someone else. These are the standard PTSD criteria where a qualifying event

"I had dissociation and in my mind, I could create imaginary friends . . . so that's what I did."

—OLGA TRUJILLO *(diagnosed with DID)*

"I could feel the world around me start spinning like a cyclone; my breathing would slow down and the world would start spinning. I knew I was going to switch and when that happened, *I* would be gone and some other part of me would be there."

—DIANNE HARPER
(formerly diagnosed with DID, now identifies as integrated although clarifies that for her it isn't either/or, "I just am who I am")

is necessary. As discussed later in the chapter, the less formally codified but immensely relevant construct of complex PTSD can get more complicated.

In DSM-5, *depersonalization* is defined as "persistent or recurrent experiences of feeling detached from, as if one were an outside observer of, one's mental process or body" (potentially an avoidance or negative mood/cognition manifestation). *Derealization* is defined as "persistent or recurrent experiences of unreality of surroundings" (potentially a part of the PTSD symptoms of intrusion, avoidance, or negative mood/cognitions).[7] Although depersonalization and derealization still appear as their own diagnoses in the dissociative disorders category, they should be ruled out if PTSD is the better explanation.

This is a gray area to navigate diagnostically, particularly because people struggling with clinically significant dissociative disorders likely meet the criteria for PTSD multiple times over. With PTSD long being conceptualized as a more event-centric diagnosis that doesn't accurately encapsulate the depth of complex trauma, this qualifier may be more appropriate for adults who experience a traumatic event not connected to childhood or developmental trauma and develop these dissociative tendencies as a result.

Complex trauma, which is now identified in the ICD-11 yet still remains absent in the DSM, can generally be described as experiences that:

- Are repetitive or prolonged
- Involve direct harm and/or neglect or abandonment by caregivers or ostensibly responsible adults

---

"Is dissociation happening in my brain or happening in my mind? Now in the present my brain is trying to decide if this is a current threat or if this is from before; but the mind is a lot more colorful. It's not *scientific*. It's a buffet of interpersonal choice."

—AMY WAGNER
(diagnosed with DID, now identifies as having a dissociative experience of life)

"I honestly don't feel I have a body at that point when I separate. I feel that freeze and anything else that happens is not me."

—KATHARINE
(identified as having DID, officially diagnosed with PTSD)

- Occur at developmentally vulnerable times in the victim's life, such as early childhood
- Have great potential to severely compromise a child's development[18]

Twenty of our contributors specifically identified complex trauma, sometimes called CPTSD, as one of their primary clinical presentations and identified experiencing a significant amount of dissociation as part of their CPTSD, even though they don't specifically identify as having a dissociative disorder. And many of these contributors with CPTSD also identify as having other diagnoses like eating disorders, substance use disorder, or forms of neurodivergence (e.g., ADHD, autism spectrum disorder) that will be more fully explored in the next section.

Fiona* is a gender-fluid clinical mental health therapist from the United Kingdom who describes herself/themselves as having had the stereotypical complex trauma narrative growing up, commenting, "I tick a majority of the Adverse Childhood Experiences (ACE) questionnaire." Fiona spent her adolescence in and out of various levels of mental health care, being treated for every possible diagnostic label she could be given, yet it wasn't until she was eighteen that she began on a treatment path that helped her understand

---

* Pseudonym given to a participant who wishes to remain anonymous.

"It's a narrowing of attention like in a tunnel and I can see just a little bit ahead (like a trance). In a parts switch, even though I am co-conscious the majority of the time, it's having the urge to do something different but not being able to stop myself."

—CHRISTY DUNN (*diagnosed with DID*)

"If I had to simplify it, in OSDD alters can and often are present, but the primary experience of dissociation is not switching. OSDD is 'light'; DID is everything turned up to eleven. However, OSDD can be covert longer."

—A.J. (*diagnosed with OSDD and later with concurrent ADHD*)

trauma at its core. Although she was given an unspecified dissociative disorder diagnosis at that point, she believes that seeing herself as having complex trauma with dissociation works better for her. In her estimation, the dissociative disorders can still bring up a connotation of "your personality is damaged," and other old hangovers of meaning from when complex trauma was labeled as hysteria, especially in women. Fiona was one of our contributors who directly asserted "I am not Sybil" in her interview. Fiona also identifies a sense of dysphoria that accompanies being gender-fluid; they report that this dysphoria is not constant, rather comes and goes. They also have a history of being treated for substance misuse and codependency, primarily using 12-step models for that treatment.

Fiona's description of all of the phenomena that we've discussed in this chapter is very detailed as it relates to her lived experience, and many of these themes and concepts also resonate from the sharing of other contributors who also identify as having dissociation as part of their complex trauma. She reflects:

Dissociation is a sense of being off-kilter somewhere inside, something not quite where it should be. A subtle shift begins when there is an emotional flashback, that some part of me is somewhere else. If I don't get that piece back in place, the lens through which I see the world is distorted and I pick up more triggers, more distress; my sleep goes and then I can be overtired and pick a fight with a partner, and it escalates to the point where now many pieces are out of place but not just one and I'm pulled in 2–3 different directions at the same time even though I'm here and appear to be going about as normal. On the more extreme end of this, the emotion "deadens" and the world is hostile, people are threatening. I become afraid to make contact with other people and it feels unsafe inside and inside becomes scary. Then I try doing things to comfort that (e.g., overeating). Not like I want to overeat, I just find myself doing that. At this level it's quite subtle: "I'm doing things but it doesn't feel like it's really me." There's a sense of increasing separation from the self, can no longer discern safety from danger, things take on a filmic quality. Physical numbing, physical pain . . . can get kind of hollow.

Please see "In Their Own Words" on page 64 for other descriptions of how contributors who primarily identify with the CPTSD or complex trauma framework explain their experiences of dissociation.

Intersections

Since my early days as a teacher in the field, I've cautioned my students about the precarious nature of Western mental health diagnosis. There are so many symptom clusters that can fit into a variety of diagnoses within the DSM, which can often lead to people being misdiagnosed—especially if the practitioner is primarily medication-focused and doesn't adequately understand dissociation or trauma. That was clearly the experience of many of our contributors. The most relevant word to emerge from the interviews is that of *intersections*—challenging us to consider how two or more diagnoses existing together may create their own set of issues, identity struggles, or perhaps even gifts. Although fundamentally a different construct, there are some similarities to *intersectionality,* a social justice framework that we discuss further in chapter 5.

While we've established that a form of dissociation can show up in all mental health diagnoses, we must also center in on the experience of people who identify having a dissociative disorder and/or dissociation present as part of complex trauma *and* another diagnosis or series of diagnoses. Many of the contributors we've featured thus far in the book spoke to their intersections, yet this section emphasizes some contributors who specifically spoke to their diagnostic intersections. For them understanding the subtle differences between each diagnosis and learning to realize how they interplay with each other is an important component of their healing process.

In Their Own Words: CPTSD

On the experiences of dissociation within complex trauma, here are some offerings from our contributors:

"There are two sides of me. One is the not changing side: my essence, the earliest memory of that was early childhood. Free, inquisitive, curious. This is the *sky,* the backdrop that's always been there. Then there's the side of me that has formed through challenges of life, which has left me cut off from the essence. When you're not living in the essence, you're in struggle."   —MALIKA

"The brain feels like everything shuts off."   —DANYALE WEEMS

NEURODIVERGENCE

The social psychologist Judy Singer coined the term *neurodiversity* in 1998, referring to nonpathological differences in the brain that contribute to difficulties with learning, mood management, attention, and other mental functions.[19] Neurodiversity generally resists a narrative that people struggling with these issues need to be cured or fixed. Neurodiversity also emphasizes that societal barriers are the greatest factor to receiving good mental health care, more so than anything inherently pathological. Though not without controversy, the autism communities and those with attention deficit-hyperactivity disorder (ADHD) have most strongly adopted use of the term. While people with other traditionally conceptualized mental health disorders, including those with dissociative disorders, see the term as applying to them, the general consensus is that dissociative disorders in and of themselves do not meet the description of *neurodivergence.*

Erin, a clinical social worker and trauma specialist treated for both ADHD and dissociation as part of her complex trauma history, offers some clarity on what can make neurodivergence and dissociative processes different, and how they inevitably interplay. Erin begins by offering her description of how dissociative symptoms developed for her as part of complex trauma:

> My experience of dissociation has been emotional numbness and detachment since I grew up in a house without emotional validation and attachment. It was an addictive household. There was a lot of ignoring of what's going on,

---

"I feel like I'm in an imaginary place. It feels like I'm not in my body and not in my brain. My brain is in this other place being happy in the characters of a book or on the Internet just learning."

—RACHAEL

"When I finally fell into my body, I fell into everything I had pushed aside."   —THOMAS ZIMMERMAN

"I'm not a diagnosis anymore, I am just *me*. In science there is no in between. Science is black-and-white and the world is full of color."

—CRYSTAL

Irish Catholic values, burying shame in alcohol that was also intergenerational. This set the stage for me to ignore and to block out other things, it fueled presentation of anxiety and somatic distress and over time created a lot of maladaptive coping.

In Erin's experience, learning to treat the dissociation components of complex trauma then led to a flare-up in what was diagnosed as ADHD. This phenomenon makes sense to her because looking back over the course of her life, she is now able to identify attention deficit issues that were there before the onset of her biggest traumatic experience.

In Erin's experience, she notices that traditional grounding skills tend to help with the lack of presence she experiences connected to dissociation and distress in her parts system. When her lack of presence is attention-related, moving and fidgeting seem to help the most. She also notes that ADHD symptoms can more randomly creep in, whereas she is eventually able to trace dissociative responses to some kind of trauma trigger. Erin affirms that the combination of trauma-focused psychotherapy and medication management (for the ADHD) are essential to her overall well-being and functioning.

Chuck Bernsohn, whom we met in the previous chapter, identified the intersection of their transgender identity and chronic pain as a dysphoria that lends itself to a high potential for dissociation. Add to the mix Chuck's attention deficit disorder (ADD) diagnosis, and some new layers of

---

"It's like there is a buffer and a barrier between me and everything else. There is a distortion in the space-time continuum. The more somatic work that I do, the more I am able to bring the two together. Because of the somatic work I haven't experienced 'leaving' in that way in a long time."

—SUNNEE HOPE

"The physical pain creates what feels like a TV static. I can dissociate to the point where I am catatonic and my brain knows that I need to move, but my body cannot move. There is an overall numbing of everything."

—JACQUELINE LUCAS

complexity are introduced. Chuck notes that it took receiving this diagnosis of ADD to realize that it could be physically painful to focus—which they believe is why they struggle with object permanence, short-term memory, rejection-sensitive dysphoria, and much anxiety weaving through all of these points of intersection.

Katarina Lundgren, the Swedish equine therapist we met in the introduction, has long been aware of her DID, identifying over two hundred parts (some she describes as fragments now, and about twenty-five are active currently). She sees herself as "not disorganized, rather, differently organized; not disordered; just differently ordered." Katarina recently confirmed her suspicion that she also has autism spectrum disorder (ASD). She feels that her autism made her more susceptible to developing DID when she was exposed to complex trauma, and she would like to see further research into this area in the years to come.[20]

Of her lived experience, Katarina offers:

> Autism can be described as a way of not tolerating the world. So there needs to be a shut-down mechanism (or shut-out). The world hurts too much . . . so there is a lot of dissociation to deal with overwhelm but also masking and using personas. So what happens if a person with high autistic traits (hyperfocused, hyperemotional, hyper-sensitive, with hyper-memory) is severely abused? Then there would be even more dissociation, identity confusions (which is also common in autism—like asking—who am I?), more depersonalization and derealization (due to overwhelm), more panic in the system. I think we need to look at who develops DID not only out of how severe the trauma is—but also who the person is behind the trauma. DID explains me to a certain degree—but learning more about autism—it really makes me see me. It is super hard. I cry a lot. But I am finally and slowly coming home.

EATING DISORDERS AND ADDICTIONS

Coming home to one's body is described by many of our contributors as a fruit of their recovery from addictions (many of which were covered earlier in this chapter) and eating disorders. While trauma-focused eating disorder treatment often parallels care for trauma-focused addiction treatment, there are some unique elements to eating disorders that several of our contributors speak to. In chapter 1, Elizabeth Davis (my personal therapist) addressed how her eating disorder was a way to escape her body that was ravaged by Major Depression. Holli Ellis, who identified as "a therapist by training, a trauma survivor by life," reports an eating disorder in her past and complex trauma with dissociative features; yet in the medical system was really only treated for Generalized Anxiety Disorder (GAD). Reflecting on her eating disorder, in the scope of her complex trauma experience, Holli described, "A big component is when I had out-of-body experiences, feeling like I was not connected to my body. In these moments I cannot connect to what people are saying."

Moreover, the disordered eating experiences of dissociation made her realize just how many blocks and chunks of her childhood may be missing. For Holli, when she dissociates, it feels like a switch has been flipped in her brain and it's a very draining experience. She continues, "I'm normally a sparkly person, like the unicorn emoji, yet when dissociation happens, it feels like the color is draining out of my soul and I go to a very shut-down place." While this can still happen to some degree in her healing, she notes that before significant treatment, a seven-year-old part would take over when this happened.

Alicia Hann is a professional dancer who also works as the executive manager of my company, The Institute for Creative Mindfulness. Alicia plays an active role in organizing the business needs that allow me the time to do a book like this, and she also felt very strongly about sharing her lived experience for the book when I put out a call for participants. Alicia has a diagnosis of OSDD as a result of complex trauma, and was previously treated inpatient on several occasions for an eating disorder (both anorexia and bulimia). For Alicia, the "thin ideal" of dance exacerbated the development of a diagnosed eating disorder, yet she believes that her issues with food would have developed regardless. She explains that for her, planning food and being consumed by it was a way to dissociate from her feelings. In reflecting on what happens in her brain during dissociation, Alicia says, "It's like I fall down a hole and am trying to fall down a hole, trying to climb out of the brain fog." Alicia also recognizes now that it was harder for the disordered eating behaviors to heal when the trauma wasn't being treated in her first attempts at healing.

BORDERLINE PERSONALITY DISORDER

Alicia, like many survivors of complex trauma, was initially—and in her view inaccurately—diagnosed with Borderline Personality Disorder (BPD). The label of any personality disorder at one time (and sadly in many circles still does) carried a great deal of shame due to the implication that personality issues are more ingrained and thus harder to treat. Some of the common symptoms of BPD include instability in relationships and mood, vacillating between extremes of valuing and rejecting someone, binary thinking, and exposing oneself to self-destructive behaviors. However, a more trauma-focused view of personality disorders, which is fortunately coming into wider acceptance, is that personality disorders—especially Borderline Personality Disorder—are really just a manifestation of complex developmental trauma.

One of our contributors, TaNiya, directly identifies as having both a BPD and a DID diagnosis, actively describing herself as having one foot in one diagnosis, and the other foot in the other. She describes an extensive history of complex developmental trauma, being incarcerated as early as thirteen after being raised by a narcissistic and abusive mother. TaNiya's issues with alcohol, other substances, and what she describes as "putting myself in bad situations" started around that age as well. TaNiya describes herself as a very loud person, and her system (which contains a strong persecutor part, or introject) can amplify this loudness. She believes this loudness is because her mother always tried to physically restrain her from speaking.

In reflecting upon the interplay between her two major diagnoses, she sees the BPD as largely being responsible for her black-and-white thinking, social paranoia, and doing everything in relationships and interactions to avoid abandonment. With the DID, she notices that her mother has a tendency to come out, due to the strong persecutor part within her system. There are other parts that were pushed and tortured so far to survive, and they are still there. Yet she also describes her system as very "stubborn and smart."

TRAUMATIC BRAIN INJURIES

A final area of intersection where we had multiple contributors comment is related to traumatic brain injuries. Amy Brickler, a therapist who initially took an extended leave after her DID was diagnosed in order to properly learn about her system, has always been fascinated by how the brain works, and not just because of her DID. Amy was born with hydrocephalus (an abnormal collection of cerebral spinal fluid in the brain) and Dandy-Walker Syndrome (a rare condition in which the cerebellum, linking the right and left hemispheres, does not fully form). She says with an air of humor, "If you look at a CT or MRI scan of my brain, it's basically underwater. So much fluid."

Amy said that as a kid, every odd thing she did was chalked up to the hydrocephalus or the Dandy-Walker Syndrome—although looking back now, many of those symptoms were dissociative in nature. Like Katarina, our contributor with autism spectrum disorder, Amy does wonder if the way she was born made her more vulnerable to developing dissociative symptoms as a response to complex trauma. For her, dissociation is like getting sucked into another world. Even though she has a very differentiated system, she does not identify switching between parts as much, yet they can all get sucked in and out of whatever this other world is. Interestingly, the metaphor that Amy uses to describe her system is a galaxy.

Sarah Smith is a practicing therapist in long-term recovery (over thirty years) from alcohol and heroin addiction. During an assault she endured when she was in active addiction, Sarah developed a traumatic brain injury (TBI) that continues to cause her problems to this day. Sarah came of age in an era when "you didn't talk about trauma in recovery," so she believes that much of what she came to learn about herself as being more aligned with a dissociative disorder was only ever labeled as depression. However, being able to work at this stage of her life with a therapist who understands Addiction as Dissociation has facilitated a new era of growth and connection.

Sarah, who saw her addiction as a way to dissociate, shares, "When I got sober thirty-one years ago, it ripped the Band-Aid off. If I didn't have all the parts holding the different memories, I couldn't have stood it."

In reflecting on her TBI, resulting from the sexual assault of which she has no memory, Sarah continues, "It feels like a part of me did die, that part isn't there anymore. It impacts my personality, impacts coping. A piece of me that's never going to be safe." She strongly agrees with recommendations made by Steele, Boon, and van der Hart in their 2017 book *Treating Trauma-Related Dissociation: A Practical, Integrated Approach.* They note that "it is essential to assess for traumatic brain injury (TBI) in patients who have been chronically abused since childhood or have a history of physical assault or accidents potentially resulting in head injury. Undiagnosed and untreated TBI can significantly interfere with therapy progress."[21]

Sarah says it's very sad when she considers that this is a part of her that can't be reached, no matter how hard others may try. And even though she states that she has been successful in both her recovery and her career, it can be a constant struggle at times, especially with organizational skills and other tasks. In further reflecting on TBI, Sarah asserts that it is important to acknowledge that a part or parts of them were lost and to acknowledge any grief or shame around how the injury may have happened (especially for those in addiction recovery). This acknowledgment may be some of the most valuable *parts work* that you do with people like Sarah. You'll read more about working with your parts in chapter 4.

We Exist—Even amidst the Controversies and Myths

While the myths and controversies surrounding dissociation and dissociative disorders will be fully unpacked in our chapter on removing stigma (chapter 7), it bears acknowledgment here that they exist. There are so many professionals I've worked with over the years, leaders I've heard speak, and writers I've read who might read the lived experience that our contributors share in this chapter and laugh. As Dr. Paul Miller recalls—whose explanations about the neuroscience of dissociation helped illuminate this chapter— at the time he began his work investigating psychosis as a dissociative phenomenon in the 1990s, many in Northern Ireland didn't even believe in dissociation. He recalls hearing a prominent psychiatrist interviewed who said that to diagnose DID, you just need a "plausible patient and a gullible psychiatrist."

Sandra (Zuleikha) Johnson, a working psychotherapist, was first diagnosed with DID in the 1980s. She currently works as part of a mental health system in a large American city where one of the two psychiatrists on site doesn't believe in dissociation.

"He believes we're all making it up," she says.

Sandra is a survivor of complex trauma and identifies ritual Satanic abuse and mind control as part of her story. Sandra acknowledges that many people, even prominent people in the field, don't believe in it, but she has had her experience verified by other people and other therapists in her area and she reports that's all the validation that she needs. When she was first diagnosed, there was a great deal of interest in her city about dissociation and trauma, and then all of a sudden, there seemed to be a backlash. She recalls that one of the prominent dissociative specialists in her area got sued by the family members of that therapist's patient, who accused the family of abuse. This made everyone scared to even approach anything with dissociation or multiplicity, a common controversy in the "memory wars" that we explore more fully in chapter 7. Sandra is grateful that her long-term therapist did not cut off this aspect of their work although reports that the entire experience "was awful to go through. It felt like such a betrayal by the mental health system."

Our hope is that one day people with dissociative disorders, dissociative minds, dissociative experiences of life, or dissociative coping mechanisms will be taken seriously and seen as they truly are—as survivors of and most often thrivers in this dance of life. To answer the question that opens this chapter, there may be some interesting things going on in your brain, but we truly believe that there is nothing wrong with you. Being human is a challenging experience, especially as people continue to mistreat and abuse each other, often as a result of their own unhealed trauma playing out in the world. Taking trauma, dissociation, and its various manifestations seriously is critical as we learn to care for ourselves, even if others have made you feel like your trauma and how you cope with it isn't valid. We hope that some of the ideas and voices in this chapter have helped acknowledge that what you may be experiencing is very real. You are indeed worthy and deserving of your story and your lived experiences being taken seriously.

EXPRESSIVE ARTS PRACTICE: INTERSECTIONS

If you think back to your early years in school, you may remember creating a Venn diagram, or presentation of shapes (most commonly circles) that intersect at certain points of commonality. You can search "Venn diagram" on your favorite Internet search engine to see some examples. The coloring page that accompanies this chapter also gives you an example of a Venn diagram.

In this expressive arts practice, you are invited to create your own Venn diagram that would give someone who is trying to get to know you—whether that be a friend or a helping professional—an idea about your diagnostic or symptomatic points of intersection or overlap. As it relates to this chapter, you can visually depict—using as many colors or shapes as you want—how diagnoses you may have received or symptoms you may have experienced (or still experience) overlap. You can even do what some of our contributors do and describe in plain language what's going on in your brain and body when you experience symptoms of dissociation, and note how they overlap and interplay. Perhaps you'll also bring in some shapes or colors to represent other aspects of your identity that are important to you such as your sexual orientation, gender identity, ethnic or racial background, education, birthplace, and spiritual or religious affiliations. We will explore some of these other areas of identity as we discuss intersectionality in chapter 5, although you are free to start brainstorming about them now. I truly invite you to bring this Venn diagram to life!

This is your creative expression, so there is no wrong way to do this practice. If you are currently engaged with a psychotherapist, a helping professional, or are part of a communal support group, consider sharing this expression with them.

═QUESTIONS TO ASK YOUR THERAPIST OR PSYCHIATRIST═

- (Assuming you established in the introduction questions with your provider whether they recognize the existence of dissociation): Has there ever been a time in your career when you had doubts? What helped you work through those doubts?

- What do you see as the difference between the brain and the mind?

- What do you believe is happening in the brain or mind of someone who dissociates? Is it just one thing for you, or do you see it as a combination of processes?

- What is your approach to diagnosis?

- Do you believe that diagnoses can change and evolve over time?

- How do you work with two or more diagnoses existing together at the same time?

- What limitations do you see in the DSM and Western psychology and psychiatry overall? Are you open to other paths of inquiry, such as Indigenous approaches to healing?

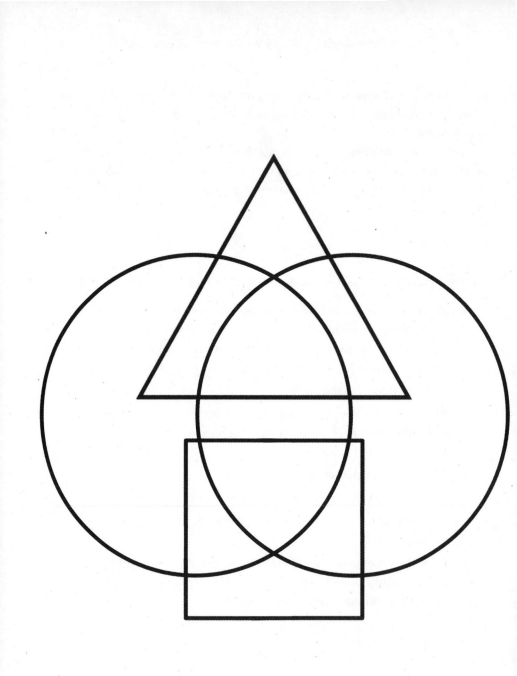

How to Build Grounding and Safety Skills (When You're Used to Escaping the Moment and Not Being Safe)

*Do not try to save the world or do anything grandiose.
Instead, create a clearing in the dense forest of your life and
wait there patiently until the song that is your life falls into
your own cupped hands and you recognize and greet it.*

—MARTHA POSTLEWAITE

In most clinical trainings on working with dissociation, teachers emphasize the importance of being able to get clients *grounded*. The practice of grounding, which can fall under the umbrella of mindfulness-informed interventions, is so widely used by clinical professionals these days, its meaning can get lost. Or many therapists will work with their clients on "grounding" and "mindfulness" skills without the client fully understanding what these skills are and why they matter for healing and recovery. Moreover, I see a large problem with therapists and other helping professionals reading these skills out of a workbook or popping on a YouTube video of a meditation for their clients, without stopping to consider how difficult it can be for a client who struggles with dissociation to even consider being mindful.

Because in many ways, the act of dissociation can be viewed as the opposite of mindfulness.

If dissociation is about escaping the present moment because the present moment is unpleasant, overwhelming, or otherwise painful, mindfulness—according to its Sanskrit word origin, *smriti*—is about remembering that you were once aware and you are now deliberately returning to that present-moment awareness. Christine Forner, a scholar, conscious practitioner, and past president of the International Society for the Study of Trauma and Dissociation (ISSTD), posits that mindfulness is fundamentally about connection (e.g., to the self, to the present moment, to others), whereas dissociation is ultimately about surviving disconnection.[1] Thus, if a person dissociates long enough or becomes bonded to this state, they can become phobic of mindfulness.

If dissociation has been your baseline way of coping, I recognize how difficult it can be for you to practice mindfulness, specifically the skill that we might call grounding. It can be even more difficult to cultivate a set of resources that help you feel some sense of internal safety. You also may have experienced a phenomenon that many of our contributors describe, which is the ability to be both present/mindful *and* dissociated at the same time (i.e., one foot in the present, and one foot somewhere else). And people who work with you therapeutically may have difficulty framing this experience.

The general consensus in treatment standards for working with both complex trauma and dissociative disorders is that developing a set of skills for coping, stabilizing, grounding, or returning to the here and now is a vital part of the process. These skills can help you explore your own relationship with safety, especially within yourself, which can be very important before you go into deeper aspects of your healing work. Our contributors were happy to share in their interviews what has worked for them in this process. We will begin by unpacking the definition of *grounding* (and offering viable alternatives if this word doesn't work for you), and then explore specific methods for grounding and how to implement them based on the lived experience of our contributors. We will come in with a section of commentary on the best strategies for both trauma-informing and dissociation-informing grounding and mindfulness practices. The chapter then concludes with a discussion on what safety may or may not mean to you and why this matters to your healing process.

Grounding: Meanings and Layers

Before reading on in this chapter, you may pause for a moment and reflect on what *grounding* means to you, or how you might define it based on your own lived experience.

Again, I am not looking for an academic definition. Notice what your body might give you instantly as an answer and then contemplate that for a moment.

The general definition that I teach for *grounding* in my clinical courses is a combination of spiritual director Martha Postlewaite's work on grounding[2] with some of my own flair added in. *Grounding is using any and all available senses and experiences to remain in the present moment, or to return to the present moment.* I emphasize to my students and clients that wandering away from present-moment awareness is normal for any human being. And when dissociation is in play as a preferred or even automatic coping skill for you, wandering is expected.

As a mindfulness meditation facilitator and therapist who teaches her fair share of grounding to people, I want you to know that whenever you try a new strategy like grounding or any other meditation or coping technique, it's going to be normal for your concentration and attention to wander. No one expects you to get it the first time. Moreover, I've been practicing meditation for most of my adult life and even to this day when I practice, my attention will wander. These practices are never about how long you can stay mindful or quiet, they are really about how you are able to use them to return to the present moment, or sense of groundedness, once you realize that you (and if it applies, your internal system) may have wandered away. Whenever I set up a mindfulness skill during a course, I always tell my students, "For the next few minutes we're going to get quiet. Even if your attention wanders eight, ten, or twenty times in a minute, it does not mean that you have failed mindfulness. The real practice is in the returning once you recognize that you may have drifted away."

Taking it a step further—even the recognition that your attention or conscious awareness may have drifted away is still a mindfulness practice! Recognizing that you are not fully present is arguably the most difficult mindfulness practice of all. And your willingness to show up and give these skills a try is the brave beginning to developing a practice that works for you.

In keeping with the definition that I proposed in this section, it's also important to emphasize that grounding and the larger sphere of mindfulness practice does *not* automatically mean seated meditation. I am the first to recognize how sitting in stillness and being quiet might be overwhelming for any trauma survivor who has been accustomed to dissociating from their feeling states. For John Fugett, a mental health therapist with a long history of being diagnosed with everything *but* a dissociative disorder, attempting these sitting mindfulness practices was just an invitation to dissociate longer and deeper!

So even though learning how to meditate quietly in a seated posture might become an important part of your healing, please know that you never have to start there. You'll discover in the next section how many of our contributors actively ground using a variety of activities and practices. In my work as a mindfulness teacher, I've long been inspired by this teaching from a ninety-eight-year-old Chan master, as delivered to Jon Kabat-Zinn (the developer of Mindfulness-Based Stress Reduction and considered by many to be the father of modern secular mindfulness). The master offered, "There are an infinite number of ways in which people suffer. Therefore, there must be an infinite number of ways in which Dharma* is available to people."[3]

Before we begin our deep dive into listening to specific methods and practices offered by our contributors, we first want to recognize that the word *grounding* may not be the best fit for you. In my view, trauma-informing anything means that we can always modify our language if we need to, especially if it makes trying out a new skill or approach more accessible to you. For Destiny Aspen Mowadeng, whom we've met in previous chapters, the word *grounding* does not work for her, especially as someone who spends her life in a wheelchair. She prefers instead the word *anchoring*, because it doesn't make her feel as stuck, punished, or trapped. Destiny also likes the concept often used in dialectical behavior therapy of *riding the wave* of experience. I often use this phrase in the various venues where I teach mindfulness strategies and yoga as it is a useful reminder to us that at its core, mindfulness is not merely a relaxation technique. Mindfulness is about being with or returning to whatever the present moment brings

---

* This is one of those words where there is not an easy translation into Western languages. "Righteousness" and "truth" are common attempts. In my work I generally define *dharma* as "the universal truths or teachings that lead us to righteousness and goodness."

us. We can ride the wave of that experience, and enough practice can teach us that when we can metaphorically surf or swim, the wave is not going to engulf us.

For Chuck Bernsohn, who earlier offered their lived experience about living with chronic pain and a disability, the word *settling* is another viable alternative in the English language. Chuck also wants to communicate that getting comfortable might not be realistic in any mindfulness, meditation, or grounding strategy for people with chronic pain, so they use the language for themselves of "get as comfortable as you can" and they encourage therapists or others teaching mindfulness to consider a similar strategy.

Before moving on, perhaps take a minute and reflect on or write down, uncensored, other terms that might work for you besides *grounding*. It may be more helpful to first read through the ideas and insights on how contributors work through struggles. Also bear in mind that if you identify as having a parts system, some parts in your system may like the word *grounding* and others might not. It's more than okay to have several different words or concepts in play.

Also consider that you and your system (if you identify one) do not need to ground perfectly, and different opinions might emerge on what constitutes grounding or similar constructs. When contributor Amy Wagner was asked the question about grounding, one of her parts chimed in and said, "You were never grounded, you were a hot air balloon." Amy laughed and recognized how much has evolved and changed for her (and the system) over the years. Still, be prepared to engage in some play with what your system has to say about all of this as you explore what it means to find your grounding, anchoring, footing, settling, etc.

101+ Ways to Ground

I've learned many different strategies for grounding in my over twenty years of pursuing healing and recovery. I also teach EMDR Therapy, yoga, and various forms of meditation . . . and I am still constantly on the lookout for new strategies I can share with my clients and students about how to most effectively ground. So I was delighted to obtain even more ideas from our contributors from a variety of different healing systems, paths, and traditions. We truly hope that one or more of these strategies—including some of the insights on how respective contributors implemented them—will be useful to you as you consider ideas for how to work with grounding, anchoring, or whatever word you choose that suggests using any and all experiences and senses to remain connected to (or return to connection with) the present moment.

Before going into the specific categories of practice that unfolded in response to the question, "What are the most effective skills you've developed for yourself in order to keep yourself grounded or safe enough?" I want to feature a sharing from contributor Dr. Kellie Kirksey on why she finds grounding necessary for health. Dr. Kellie, an African American therapist and facilitator of African-centered healing practices, is one of the most dynamic and real educators that I know. Dr. Kellie grew up in inner-city Cleveland, Ohio in a home that did not necessarily feel safe, and she was constantly finding ways to escape—both adaptive (dancing and drumming) and maladaptive (overworking). Dr. Kellie, who speaks actively on the impact of institutional and structural racism and how she continues to feel unsafe in America as a Black woman, describes that for her dissociation is what African Americans are expected to do in order to "play nice" in dominant culture.

Says Dr. Kellie, "Black Americans have been dissociating since slavery began."

Dr. Kellie sees grounding as a nourishing practice that helps us come back to the essence of who we really are, not just something that is a prerequisite for deeper healing to happen later. For Dr. Kellie, grounding brings her back to that nourishment and sense of safety within herself, which is imperative for surviving a world that is still fundamentally unsafe for her. As a deeply spiritual person, grounding practices like drumming and dancing open her up for a larger, healing spiritual connection to take place.

You many notice in the categories that follow that there is overlap or intersection. For instance, some of the practices that we've categorized under multisensory strategies may also apply to being in nature, and practices in many categories may also qualify under spiritual practice. As with many elements addressed in this book, precise categorization is impossible. We did our best here to give you some kind of structure to consider the general ways in which grounding and mindful connection may be attainable to you. We have listed the categories going from the greatest number of responses from contributors per category down to the fewest. You don't necessarily have to read into this choice since this is about quality over quantity, although we thought you might like to know which areas of practice seemed to show up the most across our contributor population.

Connecting with the Senses

Twenty-eight of our sixty-one contributors directly identified some type of practice where engaging with one or more of the five major senses helped them achieve or maintain a sense of grounding (or whatever word you may choose in its place). Some of the practices that were specifically named include:

- Essential oils and aromatherapy
- Using a cold washcloth or ice cubes/ice packs
- Alternating hot and cold temperatures
- Tossing a pillow back and forth with someone
- Tossing a ball of any texture or crumpled-up piece of paper back and forth
- Making tactile contact with a variety of objects (e.g., spiky plastic balls, mala beads, toys, rocks, recovery coins, stuffed animals)
- Gentle sounds (e.g., using an app or ringing a bell)
- Making contact with water (e.g., always having a glass of water nearby, access to a pool, other natural bodies of water or showers/baths)
- Mints and candies
- Putting feet on the ground deliberately
- Engaging in safe and appropriate touch with others
- Pushing against a wall
- Engaging with any sensation and not trying to push it away, even if that sensation is pain
- Sitting on the ground and literally touching the floor
- Sensory scanning activities or as an alternative, engaging in tasks that require one to count up or down

Several contributors mentioned the popular 5-4-3-2-1 activity. In this activity, one looks around their room to notice and name five things they see, four things they can touch, three things they hear, two things they smell, and one thing they taste. When I do this exercise with my clients I don't use the count as a hard and fast rule, rather, I have the client scan the room with all available senses and notice whatever they notice. I ask them to particularly pay attention to which two sensory channels feel the strongest for them on any given day, and perhaps to enroll those two experiences as a grounding anchor if at any time they are feeling overwhelmed, disconnected, or otherwise dissociated in a session. It can be as simple as "I see that clock on the wall," or "I can smell the orange-scented lotion on my hands" if they feel disconnected.

Two of our collaborators specifically mentioned that this skill, now a classic in dissociation-informed psychotherapy, doesn't quite work for them. Cheryl, a contributor that we first met in chapter 2, offers a viable alternative: "The five senses grounding thing doesn't really work for me but it can be helpful, especially if I'm at work, to start by naming a fruit or a vegetable that starts with A. Then B, C, etc. Singing a song like '99 Bottles of Beer on the Wall' can have a similar effect."

Many contributors noted that any contact with sensation helps them to know that they are here, now, and present. Two of the strategies offered by contributors, actually sitting down on the ground and touching it, or planting one's feet firmly into the ground, are strategies that I will use with my clients. I've done entire therapy sessions sitting down on the ground with clients if this is their wish. With the feet strategy, as long as their feet are available to do this, I will invite my clients to press their feet into the ground, look at them for a sense of visual anchoring, and then perhaps use a saying like, "My feet will not lie to me. My mind can pull me into the past or project me into the future, but my feet will always tell me where I am at in any given moment." If you do not have full access to your feet, using the hands on a table can also be a viable modification for this practice.

Several contributors noted the use of physical touch (e.g., holding a hand, cuddling, or receiving a hug), yet all noted that a safe person and context was necessary. For Crystal, the specific practice of sitting back to back with someone and having their backs make contact with each other is ideal. That way, touch and support are still received but there feels like no pressure to look at the person or talk.

Our contributors with chronic pain issues (like Crystal) or long-term illnesses expressed interesting insights about touch and sensation. For Adam O'Brien, who grew up with a debilitating skin condition and people were constantly suggesting to him what he should or shouldn't be feeling, "Pain is grounding. It allows me to know that I'm alive, otherwise, I'm numb." While I am certainly not suggesting that people deliberately inflict pain on themselves in order to ground, it can give insight into why so many of us with dissociative experiences of life have also used self-injury in order to cope. Yet what Adam seems to be suggesting is that if chronic pain is part of your life, learning how to be with it mindfully and not trying to push it away can become a grounding practice.

Many contributors spoke about working with ice or alternating cooling and warming experiences to create some type of intense sensation that they can find grounding or comforting. Contributor Jacqueline Lucas offers, "Temperature control can be helpful yet difficult because of my fibromyalgia. It's not uncommon for me to sleep with both a heating pad and an ice pack."

When Jacqueline shared this, I nodded my head in recognition. I am typically that person who is driving my actual car with the air-conditioning blasting and the seat warmers on; both create a unique sensation that keeps me grounded. On many evenings during my unwinding—remember, as I'm on my couch with the cat watching TV?—it's not uncommon for me to be laying my head on an ice pack while I am underneath blankets in front of the fireplace. I often go to sleep underneath a pile of comforters and blankets while also using an ice pack as the fan whirls overhead.

Activities of Daily Living

Twenty-six of our contributors described how they turn activities of daily living around their home space into mindfulness practices, or deliberately engage certain practices as part of their daily routines to stay grounded. These responses correspond to an idea I've taught my clients and students for many years—any human activity can be turned into an opportunity to mindfully connect with the here and now. If you don't think you can sit down and deliberately meditate, what is a task you do in your daily life that you can make an effort to engage in with full attention? Some of those tasks show up on this list from our contributors:

- Taking a shower
- The entire morning routine (e.g., bathroom, getting ready, coffee, breakfast)
- Paying attention to anything one is doing at the moment
- Putting things in one's path during the day that help them feel regulated and grounded
- Gardening
- Cooking

- Paying attention to nourishing nutrition
- Cleaning
- Farm or stable tasks
- Reading
- Watching a movie (especially a kid's movie for the little parts)
- Talking out loud
- Reciting prayers, mantra, or sayings
- Staying busy (in an adaptive way)
- Going on one's cellphone or social media (in as adaptative a way as possible)

While this category may be one of the more self-explanatory ones, I'd like to bring forward statements from several of our contributors on how they might use these strategies as part of their daily routine. For sunnEe hope, "Talking out loud to myself is very orienting. To hear myself say: 'I am 55 years old and today is. . . .'" Contributor Christy Dunn, a therapist with DID, shared that throughout her day, "In coming back to reality, it helps to ask what is true and what is real."

Several contributors identify how staying busy around the house and in their life keeps them from dissociating in an unhelpful way. Everyone who shared on this does recognize how keeping busy can easily become maladaptive for them, as can going on the cellphone or social media. As described by one of our anonymous contributors, "I stay busy, I read, and prepare for my work. It helps me to have a focus. It's not where I want to be forever as a way to ground. It's not necessarily the healthiest but it's healthier than a lot of other things."

Expressive Arts (Music, Visual Art, Movement, Dance, Writing)

The expressive arts were certainly my first love and proved to be a helpful and adaptive coping device growing up in my house. I fortunately had access to dance and music lessons, and later I actively participated in speech and drama. I believe that the reason I was able to embrace my recovery and healing journey so fully in my early twenties, which included feeling the strong feelings required in that process, is because expressive art forms gave me a safe enough container for feeling feelings.

The twenty-seven participants who spoke about the role of expressive arts in their healing process did so with great enthusiasm. Some of the specific practices named include:

- Listening to music
- Playing or creating music (e.g., drumming, playing the guitar, singing, DJ-ing)
- Dance and movement
- Arts and crafts
- Doodling
- Meme-making
- Sand-tray work
- Writing
- General expressive arts practice (by therapeutic definition, working with all of the creative forms in conjunction)

A few memorable insights from our contributors speak to the healing and grounding power of expressive arts, especially in navigating life with a system, or navigating tricky places where expression can be adaptive or maladaptive. The Garden System shared with enthusiasm, "When we can't talk, we draw pictures!" Heather (LS) Scarboro+, whom we first met in the introduction, is a professionally trained musician and avid practitioner of the expressive arts—and their system is clearly grateful for these practices. Heather (LS+) observed, "I know that whatever is happening, I just pick up my guitar and play it, and everything kind of mellows out. Yet Sid, our ten-year-old's thing is art. They all have some form of a creative outlet."

For Alicia Hann, the professional dancer in recovery from an eating disorder whom we met in chapter 2, "Movement can be safe and grounding, but can be used to push away things too. I do my best to embrace a *Dancing Mindfulness** position of using the movement to embrace whatever may come, resting into feeling and changes in the body." Alicia hits on an important point: many of these expressive practices can become a doorway into dissociation too, especially if we use them to push away what we are experiencing instead of using them to help us be present with the experience of life. Learning to

---

* The specific practice system of Dancing Mindfulness developed by the author that Alicia also teaches. For more information, please go to www.dancingmindfulness.com.

engage with this mindful intention can be a process for certain if, for instance, dance, music, or art has been an escape more so than a trusted friend. Kathleen, a retired preschool teacher with DID, reports that for her the combination of music and movement helps her to ground herself and find herself, expressing, "There is healing in music and movement."

Yoga, Embodiment, Breathing, and Energy Skills

Twenty contributors directly named yoga as a specific movement practice they engage in for grounding and as a support to their recovery. Many others identified other physical practices and exercise that help them to stay grounded, with the following practices named specifically: kickboxing, outdoor workouts in the park, bike riding, running, weightlifting, playing hockey, using the punching bag, ping-pong, and tennis. Although many people in the West see yoga as "exercise," it is truly an entire system of healing that traces back to ancient India, predating the religious traditions of Hinduism and Buddhism. In modern times, yoga can mean a spiritual system for study, a physical practice, a meditative experience, an energy cleanser, and a model for working effectively with the breath.

One of our contributors, Paula S., a complex trauma survivor who works as both a therapist and a yoga teacher, speaks to the differences in practice: "The style of yoga I practice will be different depending on how my nervous system is. Because ultimately the purpose of grounding is to feel as comfortable as I can within my body in order to regulate my nervous system. My go-to, weekly ritual is to do two classes on a Thursday, first a *vinyasa* (more vigorous) and then a *yin* (gentler practice). I will do some basic yoga during the week, anything that is holding/strengthening and stabilizing."

Several contributors specifically sing yoga's praises, especially Holli Ellis: "Yoga has been such a superpower in my recovery that my husband and I both, separately, wrote yoga into our wedding vows. He said, 'I promise to always encourage you to do yoga when a former part of yourself is showing up.'"

For Alexis, the power of yoga is that her entire system resonates with it. She offers, "The entire system loves yoga. The little parts love that some of them are animals, the older part that is more sporty likes the challenge. I feel so connected to the body when I'm doing yoga because everyone in my head likes it and they work together."

As I learned when I trained in trauma-informed yoga from Mark Lilly (the founder of Street Yoga), so many movement and breath practices within yoga can be both a trigger *and* a resource. While the benefits of yoga are becoming increasingly documented, it's important to recognize that asking a person to get into their body and connect with their breath when they've been used to dissociating can be a hard ask. And it can be overwhelming. For Thomas Zimmerman, who survived a great deal of religious trauma where he was made to believe that his body could not be trusted, "Breath was horrible for me at first and then one day I found it, not long after a training that I attended. Then I was able to slow down and I intuited my way into my breath, an entryway for slowing down."

Fiona offers this accommodation that works for her when she approaches any yoga and movement practice: "I need to come into my body in a safe way and movement and organic stretching helps. Yet I may need to start by acknowledging *I have a body* in the first place." Kylie offers a useful distinction that works for her in evaluating whether her movement practices are helpful or harmful: "When you no longer feel good about what you're doing with yoga or movement, when it's no longer relaxation, then it's time to stop. Just like you might get that icky sort of feeling when you've been using the phone as a coping skill too long."

Several other practices that incorporate subtle movement were also named, although not much extensive commentary was given on their implementation: body tapping in the tradition of emotional freedom techniques (EFT) and "butterfly" or back-and-forth bilateral tapping against the body as is used in EMDR Therapy (more to follow in chapter 6).

Being in Nature and Connecting with Pets and Animals

Sixteen contributors specifically spoke to the power of going outside or being in nature as immensely helpful to their grounding and healing. For many years as a therapist, I've observed the raw power in simply being able to go outside with a client and engage in some "walk and talk" therapy, especially when the energy or flow of the session feels stale in the office. Eleven of our contributors directly identified walking outside as a grounding practice, with three contributors each naming the importance of getting their hands in the dirt and actually touching plants (which can include literal tree hugging). For Dr. Kellie Kirksey, whose poetic reflections on grounding opened this section, "I work to be in nature in such a way that I connect to the rhythms and the songs of nature."

For Susan Pease Banitt, the therapist who would rather hang out with Shamans instead of other therapists, whom we met in chapter 1, "I have a multidimensional understanding of grounding since I literally walked on my toes the first seven years of my life. It was painful to put my feet on the ground. Grounding is about nourishing and taking care of the Earth element inside of my body. Earth energy, nourishing, mother energy." For Andrea, whom we also met in chapter 1 as she discussed her experiences with derealization, nature is her anchor to the here and now. Says Andrea about a specific practice she uses, "A lot of times after a hard day, I stand outside barefoot, or I walk to a nearby creek to engage in grounding."

Several other contributors got beautifully specific about their grounding practices that take them outside. Dianne Harper, a contributor we met in chapter 2 (diagnosed with DID and now identifying as integrated or "just me") shares, "I sit outside and I drink my coffee in the morning and I notice. Sometimes it's just paying attention to one blossom." Another contributor who wishes to remain anonymous mentioned nature, the park, and going outside in almost every answer of her interview. She offers, "My safe place is nature and the park. As soon as I enter this particular park, all of me feels settled and relaxed. The trees, the plants, the animals ask nothing of me, just to be. I feel supported and connected in a very unconditional way!"

For Blaise, the firefighter-turned-therapist we first met in chapter 1, managing the grief around the tragic death of his brother is a compounding factor in his depression recovery. Yet even the act of visiting his brother's grave has invited Blaise into a deeper sense of grounding by connecting to nature. Blaise explains, "Whenever I go to my brother's grave, I go there and I sit and cry. Yet when I'm there, I am so mindful. At the treeline I can see the whole graveyard, and the beautiful blue sky. Some days I focus on the skies, other days on the trees, other days on the dirt. And I write whatever pops into my mind."

An additional eleven contributors also speak to the power of being in contact with animals in some form. One contributor, A.J., commented on the specific value of having her service dogs (first Hugo and now Wiley) to help her manage life outside of her home. She elucidates that medication and therapy have helped her manage symptoms related to her various diagnoses (ADHD, CPTSD, depression, anxiety), but her dogs gave A.J. her life back. She continues, "Wiley knows when we're about to dissociate before we do. He gives us a tether to the world around us when we'd otherwise be totally lost." For Sandra Johnson, a therapist living with DID, her pets are also a lifeline. She offered, "My first dog Jett saved our lives so many times. We have pictures of all our dogs on the walls. That's where our biggest feeling of safety comes from."

Katarina Lundgren presently runs an international NGO educating and doing research on equine assisted interventions. And even though some of her abuse involved animals, she reports that she never feels as safe as when she's with animals, specifically horses and dogs. She says, "I feel more safe being in the middle of a herd of horses, even when I walk barefoot among them, than I do with people. Because I know the horses never would hurt me on purpose."

Spiritual and Energetic Practices

Ten contributors specifically named spiritual and energetic practices as helpful to them in the grounding process. While these outlets are explored more fully in chapter 6, which covers healing practices, some of the specific practices and insights bear mentioning here in this discussion on grounding:

- Tapping into something greater than myself
- Indigenous rituals that address the interplay between fire and water (e.g., sweat lodge or *Inipi*)
- Guided Shamanic practices
- Smudging (i.e., Native American cleansing rituals involving herbs like sage)
- Meditation
- Connection to earth as a spiritual practice
- Reiki
- Acupuncture
- Cranial Sacral Therapy (CST)
- Plant-assisted or psychedelic ceremony

For Chuck Bernsohn, participating in Native American practice as guided by an elder helps them engage in their deepest levels of healing work. Chuck reflects, "Connecting to my wisest, oldest self is grounding. They are deeply self-assured, very rooted in a spirituality that has existed longer than the physical body has existed. It's an ancient knowing. They give me a trust in self that I don't experience in my day-to-day life."

Chuck, who is white, has engaged in the practice of sweat, or *Inipi,* as guided by an elder. Brandon Spangler, a white Marine veteran who currently works as a therapist in Montana, also takes part in sweat regularly, guided by elders of the Blackfeet nation. Brandon believes so strongly in sweat, he regularly runs retreats and experiences for fellow veterans to take part in this sacred practice, which we explore more fully in chapter 6. As it directly relates to grounding, Brandon explains, "For me, the sweat lodge *(Inipi)* is visceral. You're connected to the ground when it's happening. You're literally sitting on the ground. Being led by people who have generational experience with healing trauma, that's the even bigger stuff."

Dr. Kirsten Koenig, another therapist contributor who is herself the survivor of complex trauma, is Blackfeet by birth. Kirsten was adopted by two white parents from the East Coast who deliberately hid the truth of her Native origins from her throughout her adult life. As part of her healing journey, Kirsten found it essential to reconnect with the truth of who she is, which included moving back to Montana as an adult. In sharing the many layers of her story for this interview, Kirsten reflected, "During a recent trauma when the barrel of a gun was pointed into my head, I decided that it wasn't my time to go. I was shocked into the now. Into the smudge, what's going on in my world *now?* What are my senses telling me?"

If grounding is an active practice of using all available senses and experiences to reconnect with the here and now, Kirsten's experience certainly shows how that simple practice can literally save one's life. Or at least provide us with an anchor until we are able to more fully heal and bring ourselves back to life. In Kirsten's case, connection to her spiritual practices was paramount to her rekindling the life force.

Education, Self-Study, and Support

Another category that emerged from our contributors on grounding, with ten of them mentioning tasks in this area specifically, relates to the importance of educating oneself and having a support system. Sometimes this education involves learning more about one's condition, other times it's a practice that yogis call self-study *(svadhyaya)*—for instance, identifying and exploring the source of something that was triggering. Kathleen observes, "The books give me a deeper understanding and I'm not afraid to try new things." We will engage in more practices of this nature in our chapter on the Dissociative Profile (chapter 5).

Six contributors identified making contact with their support group as vital to their grounding process with an additional two specifically crediting the existence of online support groups. On the importance of support, Katarina Lundgren simply yet elegantly describes what support means for her. Katarina says, "Get yourself a village. Have yourself a team. If you're hurt in a village, you need a village to heal as well." Dr. Paul Miller echoes the same teaching, just replacing the word *village* with *community,* and says that this teaching is a fundamental component of healing in parts psychology.

Withdrawing from External Stimuli

Seven contributors describe practices that would qualify as withdrawing from excess sensory distraction as important to their overall grounding plan. Getting enough sleep, setting boundaries, and taking a nap all fall into this category. For Megan, the paramedic with DID we met in chapter 2, "Naps are my reset button. Once I can take a nap, it quiets me down and I feel so much better." I heartily relate to Megan's experience and continue to be grateful in my recovery for the gift of short naps or simply withdrawing into quiet and stillness for about twenty minutes.

Malika, a yoga teacher and survivor of complex trauma, describes her process. She offers, "I consciously withdraw into my own space. I choose not to engage with energy that doesn't serve me. For the longest time I believed that I could only conquer the abuse if I learned to survive in it. Today I've learned that stepping away is an option. Energy follows attention. So by placing my attention elsewhere, I can redirect my energy." Contributor Melissa Parker, a therapist with DID whom we met in the first chapter, cautions us not to judge the way we may see people engage in sensory withdrawal. She notes, "Sometimes I just need to stare at the wall. Some consider this dissociative, for me it's a grounding reset."

Guided Visualizations

Seven contributors spoke to the importance of visualization work specifically in helping them be able to stay grounded. Three specifically noted that a "Calm Safe Place" style meditation works for them (bringing up a place, real or imagined, where they can go as a healing resource), while several contributors noted why such an exercise is not helpful for them as people who dissociate. Fiona, who is especially frustrated with the insistence on visualization in EMDR Therapy, expresses, "If I'm already dissociative, visualization is not going to be enough to ground me." As an EMDR trainer, I tend to agree with her. I emphasize to my own trainees that they must have more at their disposal besides visualization exercises to help clients who dissociate significantly. Dr. Curt Rounazoin, who has trained others in EMDR Therapy since close to the inception of the therapy in 1989, also commented that he rarely uses the Calm

Safe Place exercise with clients. Please review the section on sensory skills for more ideas besides visualization if you are engaged in trauma-focused therapy and your provider is insisting on visualization.

Rebecca specifically noted her frustration with the Calm Safe Place–style visualization, commenting, "Doing outside guided visualizations (e.g., Calm/Happy Place) is not helpful as I truly need to stay in the room. It is helpful to notice my intense feelings and give them an external image, like a suitcase, to realize that the fear and the anxiety is not me." Other alternatives to Calm Safe Place–style visualizations offered by our contributors include visualizations like Dial-It-Back, where you imagine that your emotional intensity is at a certain number on a volume knob—like 9—and you visualize yourself "dialing it back" to 2 or 3. Another alternative mentioned by a contributor is a Grounding Tree meditation, where one imagines they are taking on the role of a tree and feeling their roots connect into the earth. You can check out my version of this meditation as a video presentation on www.traumama desimple.com/videos.

Developing a Plan That Works for You

The various practices we covered are meant only as suggestions. Just because these skills for grounding worked for our contributors does not mean that they will all work for you, or in the same way. The experience of trauma and dissociation can be very subjective person-to-person (or system-to-system); so too is the experience of healing. As an example, while I/we personally connected with many of the skills offered by our contributors, there are several that simply do not work for us, or do not work as well as others. Moreover, some skills worked for us at earlier points in our healing journey that are no longer as effective, especially as we've picked up some new strategies along the way. Yet it feels good to have a memory of what those early skills are for my toolbox because we truly never know when something might come in handy.

At this point you may consider revisiting the *"Safe Enough" Harbor* Exercise where you are asked to start brainstorming up to one hundred skills for grounding in the introduction. After reading this chapter, are there any additional skills you forgot about that you can add to that list? Might there be any skills or grounding strategies you are inspired to try out after reading this chapter?

An important word of caution is in order here. Some of the skills uncovered in this chapter are simpler and subjectively safer to try than others. Take, for instance, pushing against a wall. That is something you can try right this moment without putting in a lot of time or effort. After every skill, you can take a pause and notice what you notice. Be aware that you may need to try it several times or over a period of time in order to be able to recognize the fullness of its impact. Even a skill like pushing against the wall may come with some trial and error. Does it feel better to push with your hands and arms, or to allow the wall to support the whole weight of your body? You may consider trying those variations now and observe what you are noticing.

Any of these skills, even something as subjectively simple as pushing against a wall, can bring up some strong sensations and feelings. Having a supportive person you can touch base with (even if that's your therapist), or being able to go to another skill to assist you in managing the feelings one skill brought up is important. Perhaps your journal that you keep for both writing and artwork can be an outlet for expressing what you observe after pushing the wall. Even if that journal serves as a container for you scribbling vigorously in red crayon, notice whatever is present for you and be kind to yourself. You may discover in the process that scribbling is a better skill for you than pushing the wall!

Other skills presented here involve more care in learning how to use them as some risks may be involved, as is the case with essential oils. For many people, using oils is a relatively harmless exploration of smelling what seems nice and noticing the impact on the body–mind complex. Yet allergic reactions may be possible with oils, and using them on parts of the body where they are not intended to be used can be dangerous. While consulting with a trained aromatherapist is advisable—if that is accessible—to fully explore optimal use, looking up some general information online can still give you the peace of mind you need. In the spirit of "don't believe every-thing you read on the Internet," we advise that you consult with several sources as sometimes information on products like oils is not properly vetted or can be influenced by the business agenda of whoever is selling the oils. An increasing number of therapists are now using oils as adjuncts to their practice and may also have good information available to you on safe, trauma-informed use.

Several other skills mentioned in this chapter, while they can be fundamen-tally wonderful at their core, may not be delivered in ways that are optimally trauma-informed. Yoga is the biggest example of the phenomenon playing out in communities. Throughout my years doing this work I've heard so many horror stories of people hearing that yoga is good for them, and they end up at a studio that is very fitness-focused, promoting a "no pain, no gain mental-ity," usually with many physical adjustments being used. Such an experience for someone who is expecting something more gentle can be jolting or even re-traumatizing. So as not to single out those practitioners and teachers of what is generally called power yoga (since an increasing number of them are becoming more trauma-informed), horrifying experiences can also happen with teachers who share a physically gentler system of yoga, yet are set in their ways about how things are supposed to be taught in a specific tradition. Issues around technique adherence, like "you must close your eyes to help you fully drop in to the meditation" are big offenders.

Also be advised that even though many yoga schools and centers purport being connected to traditional lineages from India, so many of the major lineages that now operate in the United States have been embroiled in scandal around sexual misconduct and using the spiritual teachings of yoga to silence survivors when they speak up.[4] Having been involved in one of these lineages for many years, I still highly regard the skills and opportunity to work on my own practice in a traditional context. The experience gave me an opportunity to sift through some of the last layers of my own spiritual abuse healing. Yet I was repulsed by so much of what I saw and heard in the larger community where I practiced. Throughout my time studying this lineage I often commented that I would not want a trauma survivor brand new to their healing to be exposed to many of the teachings without some kind of trauma-informed guide. And the silencing of survivors to protect the power structures that are in place is inexcusable. The yoga world, both in an India that's been influenced by Western commercialism, and in the commercialized West, is plagued with these problems. My hope is that survivors can be aware of this reality without shutting themselves off to the healing power that yoga clearly can offer.

Be on the lookout for how a studio, school, or yoga facility may present themselves online. Does their online presence suggest that they are making efforts to be more trauma-informed, or that they are open to addressing issues around social consciousness and responsibility? You may also feel better about calling a studio before checking it out in person or via online classes and asking the owner or teachers about how they handle issues like physical adjustments or allowing students to opt out of certain poses. Asking them about their approach to trauma-informed yoga or working with students struggling with mental health is also advisable. For many trauma survivors, going to a studio may feel too risky, so engaging with trauma-informed yoga videos online (there are plenty available on YouTube and on my own Trauma Made Simple site) or via apps (like Calm or Insight Timer) might feel like the safer way to dip your toe into practices. More and more trauma-focused therapists are now getting trained in some elements of trauma-informed yoga, breathwork, and meditation that they might be able to share with you as a first exposure. You can then discuss with them if checking out a class or a more formal practice will benefit your healing plan.

A final caution that we offer in this area relates to responsible engagement with Indigenous practices, so many of which came up in our contributor interviews as being vital to trauma healing. As I suggested in discussing yoga, just because a teacher is from India does not mean that the teacher is automatically enlightened and ethical. They may or may not be open to discussing how your history of trauma is affecting your ability to interact with a practice. We must be mindful of this phenomenon, even with increasing attention being paid to honoring the traditional roots and traditions of practices like yoga and meditation. There are plenty of yoga teachers in the world who are not Indian in origin, have traditional grounding in the essence of what the practices are about and their cultural context, and are also open to trauma-informing how they deliver teachings. So in looking for teachers or approaches in Eastern meditation traditions like yoga, the martial arts (with origins in Japan and China), and Buddhist meditation, you can do your homework while also learning to trust your own judgment about whether you feel safe enough with a teacher. Just because a person wears holy robes or talks in a language that sounds mystical does not automatically make them safe for you.

The same general principle applies to working with any type of Indigenous healer when engaging in practices like Shamanic journeying, sweat lodge *(Inipi)*, or smudging. Even the various Native American people I interviewed for this book have different approaches and philosophies about traditional interpretations of teachings and how they ought to be shared with the world. Roger Vielle, the Blackfeet elder we met in our previous chapters, shares that there are some Native Americans who don't think Native practices are for white people. He sees it differently, believing that these practices are meant to be shared for the healing of the world.

Being responsible with how you practice is crucial, especially if you desire to be more socially conscious. In other words, I would not advise you to look up "how to smudge" or "how to set up a sweat lodge" on YouTube, especially if the videos feature a white teacher who has not clearly explained their authority or permission to share these practices. Find a Native practitioner to study with, or even a non-Native practitioner who has an understanding of what they can or cannot teach according to their own study with elders.

If trying out some of these practices feels authentic for your healing at this point, do your homework. Much of this work can be done online or through word of mouth. For instance, I was led to my connection with Roger Vielle because my student and friend Brandon Spangler invited me to be in touch with him. When I asked Roger how non–Native American people can responsibly engage with Native American practices, he offered, "As a white person, don't give your opinions or advice about what's being done if you don't know the history or the story about it."

Roger also mentioned that, as a member of the Blackfeet nation, he would not assume to tell a member of the Nez Perce nation how to conduct their healing ceremonies. Varieties of practice and differences of opinion abound, so just be mindful of this reality as you may delve into these areas of practice. Showing the same respect you would want people to offer you and/or your system is imperative and ultimately will benefit your healing. You can decide later, or in communication with your therapist if you have one, whether what you learn from these exposures will serve your healing in the long run. Yet in the moment, respect is essential.

Trauma- and Dissociation-Informing Your Practices

Many of the meditations, visualizations, yoga experiences, or other practices that you look up online or receive from a therapist or teacher can offer precise instructions on how to practice. While you may find some of these instructions helpful as you set out to learn practices, if you find the rigidity of these instructions triggering or otherwise inaccessible, know that you can make some simple modifications that might help you feel better about sticking with the practice. These are instructions I give to my clients and students on how to deliver any strategy in a more trauma- and dissociation-informed manner. You are welcome to use these too as you trial-and-error with different exercises.

EYES CAN STAY OPEN. Many teachers and recorded exercises will advise or even command you to close your eyes. This can create a sense of claustrophobia that can induce panic or anxiety. For people who dissociate often or have dissociative disorders, keeping the eyes closed too long can break a sense of attunement to the here and now of the space you're in and promote more dissociative drift. Be aware of any teacher you encounter who says you must close your eyes. Listen for language like, "Close the eyes or keep them gently open with a soft gaze."

TIME IN THE EXERCISE IS VARIABLE.   In many traditional Buddhist meditation contexts, sitting meditations can run twenty minutes or longer, and many teachers and therapists in secular traditions will lead meditations that are the length their worksheets say they should be. For many people who have been used to dissociating, practicing this long can feel like torture. Starting with fifteen or thirty seconds of any practice is more than okay. You may or may not be able to work your way up to longer practices. You are completely empowered to alter the length of time you spend in any practice. While setting a timer for practices can be a rich part of the practice, inviting you to stay with something instead of immediately dismissing it because you are bored or activated, you are in control of how long you set that timer.

CHECK YOUR ASSUMPTIONS ON WHAT MINDFULNESS OR MEDITATION MEANS.   If you go on your favorite Internet search engine right now and type in "mindfulness," what that usually returns are pristine nature objects or people who look like fashion models sitting on a beach or a mountain with a blissed-out look as their eyes are closed and legs are perfectly crossed. I do not look like this when I practice mindfulness, neither do most of my clients and students. If you think you have to look a certain way or already be a "chill" person to meditate, you may be setting yourself up to get frustrated with the practices. Mindfulness is about being with what is—if that helps you relax or be calm, then great. Yet the fullness of the practice is so much more than that. And I tell my students all the time that I am not impressed by how long you can sit still in a practice. Rather, I am delighted when I see you notice that you've left present-moment awareness and can draw yourself back to it once you recognize that your attention drifted.

BE OPEN TO VARIATIONS IN PRACTICE.   Despite what others may tell you, sitting perfectly still for a specified length of time does not automatically lead to successful mindfulness practice. As demonstrated in this chapter, there are so many different ways to attune to present-moment awareness. Honor this human necessity of variation and modification and notice what works for you.

The Complexity of Safety

One of the reasons we encourage people who dissociate to learn grounding skills is so they can cultivate a sense of safety within themselves. Creating a safe harbor within can be essential when navigating a world that fundamentally feels unsafe. The word *safety*, like *grounding*, can be so overused in the helping professions these days that we may lose its meaning. Therapists are trained to do safety checks with their clients to assess for behaviors like suicidality, self-injury, and harm to others. In trauma-focused care, one of the first tasks that therapists are asked to engage in are building skills with their clients to assure for safety. But even as a trauma-focused therapist I can roll my eyes at this directive.

"What the hell is safety anyway?" I've heard myself ask, even muttering it to myself at trainings over the years.

After everything I've been through, how can I ever hope to be safe? And as a woman in a world still dominated by misogynistic and patriarchal systems that ignore the suffering of women, can I ever really be safe? As a queer woman whose family of origin is still largely religious, living in a country and really a world where our rights are still not secure, is safety just another illusion?

Although these questions apply to us, you may have found yourself asking similar questions, personalized to your situation and how the world tends to see you. You might get angry or even enraged with a therapist, teacher, or other helper who tells you that you are in a *safe place,* that you are *safe now,* or that you are *safe with them.* I've long taught to proceed with caution or call it out if you hear someone say this, because no one ought to be telling you what you should be feeling. The word *safety* may also be charged for you if abusers or systems you were a part of that wounded you would constantly tell you that you are/were safe with them. Cheryl, one of our contributors, has learned that feeling unsafe is the primary trigger for her dissociating in the first place. And sometimes this lacking safety and stability occurs when some meaningful change is happening in her own therapeutic process. So once again, dissociating in response to not feeling safe or safe enough ought not automatically be labeled as a bad thing.

You decide whether you are safe with a person or in a given situation or context. One hundred percent safety at all times and in all situations might be unrealistic because of how the world is and how you've experienced the world due to your trauma. Yet working toward experiencing some semblance of safety, especially safety within, can be a vital part of surviving the world and engaging in a meaningful recovery experience. Perhaps the construct of *safe enough* as described in the introduction is a workable idea for you at this time. Or perhaps you can relate to what several of our contributors noted that safety means for them—and how they've developed a working sense of it in their healing.

For Jaime Pollack, even as someone who has engaged in a great deal of her own healing work and now advocates extensively for others, safety is tricky. She explains, "I've never felt safe ever in my life. Some of that is being a survivor. Some of that is being a woman. I cannot shake that sense of being prey."

Jaime expresses that each survivor of traumatic experiences needs to identify what safety means for them, and that there can be a difference between physical and emotional safety. She indicates that as it relates to physical safety, being at home with her husband there and the alarm on does help. As it relates to emotional safety, predictability, consistency, and honesty from other people are her surest ways of experiencing pockets of safety in this world. Jaime says that even though she and her husband have been together for over twelve years, it took her awhile to truly believe that this trait about him was real.

sunnEe hope is another contributor who does not ever believe she is 100% safe. Yet learning to sink into safe moments—especially within her own body—and learning to trust her body and her intuition, are important. For Erin, who also rejects the notion of 100% safety because of the world we live in, the concept of *safe enough* works for her. Moreover, her understanding of internal safety as something you can control with your exercises and skills can help. As it relates to grounding specifically, having meaningful objects around her that she can access at any given time helps with this sense of internal attachment imperative to her sense of safety.

For several of our participants who disclosed a DID diagnosis, navigating how safe the different members of a system feel is necessary. The Garden System explains that their adult parts know things are safe but the littles don't always believe it. So giving them what they need is critical. When I first met The Garden System during our interview, Jenny, one of the youngest parts, was out front first to scope me out. Jenny needs to look for the hiding places too; even if she doesn't need them, she needs to know where they are. Katarina Lundgren believes that she is always living with some degree of unsafety and uncertainty. She notices that some of her little parts can feel safer with different people yet they are mindful that this phenomenon can reflect those parts' naiveté.

"The whole of us?" she says, "we know the world can turn upside down in one millisecond."

Rebecca used to laugh whenever she heard the "Are you safe at home?" question in the hospital, because her reality for much of her life has been that she didn't feel safe anywhere. In her recovery process, she's learned the importance of experiencing a sense of safety in her own body while also staying attuned to practicalities like knowing where the exits are. She can also find a simple self-questioning strategy helpful when she is feeling especially unsafe: "Is this a past fear or a present situation?" When it's a present situation making her feel afraid or unsafe, it's usually triggered by a past fear.

For Dianne Harper, who no longer has a DID diagnosis yet navigated it for a long time, *being safe* was something she did not know how to do before all of this work, noting her continued amazement that she survived life. A series of strategies became helpful to her. On a practical level, she began by sitting upright in a chair and learning how to contract her muscles to feel a sense of safety and presence in the body. While she noted that this worked sometimes, the constant constriction felt like she was building walls around people. She eventually learned how to trust her own gut with people and allow some of these walls to loosen and become more permeable. Having a good therapist who modeled solid boundaries (e.g., no contacting the therapist after 10 PM) while also being warm and open about her own life allowed Dianne to see that an interplay of openness and protection is possible.

For Destiny Aspen Mowadeng, because of being in a wheelchair, she recognizes that total safety isn't possible yet she works to find experiences of it in the world. She does note that for certain tasks, like doing this interview, the idea of *safe enough* just doesn't cut it. She had to feel completely safe with the interviewer. Many of our contributors noted this sense of complete safety with their guide through healing as imperative, even if they didn't experience total safety in other places in the world. Other contributors noticed that even if they have moments of feeling unsafe with a therapist, which sometimes happens on bad days or if they are transitioning into a sense of some deeper work, a skillful therapist knows how to notice this and address it with care.

Amy Wagner, who continually works to navigate her dissociative experience of life, says learning to be safe within has come in increments over the years. The more she shared segments of her trauma story and grew in the understanding and nuances of her experiences, she pieced together the tapestry of her own life and realized that she was, indeed, safe. Amy says, "Safety comes from an awareness of understanding yourself. I create my own safety."

For Katharine, a therapist with DID, the very fears about how her mind worked prevented her from feeling a sense of safety within herself. She remembers, "It wasn't safe to be inside of me for a long time because I didn't accept the dissociation, I didn't even know about it. I know I felt different, knew that there was something different inside of me that most people don't experience. In grad school, when I opened the DSM to the dissociative disorders chapter my vision would blur—my system wouldn't even let me read about it."

Katharine has moved through this fear by learning about herself and taking more risks in her healing process, especially risks about sharing about herself and her own history of addiction and dissociation. Many contributors highlighted the importance of feeling internal safety through self-acceptance and surrounding themselves with others who allow them to be their authentic selves. Holli Ellis, a contributor whose insights have appeared at several points in the book, summarizes, "Can I be myself? Does my authentic self get to show up? This is what healing is for me. Continuing to work towards living in my authentic truth."

Dr. Debbie Korn, one of our professional contributors who has a great deal to offer personally, helps us pull this all together. She believes that none of us, regardless of whether we struggle with dissociation, can feel safe all the time; it is not a constant. Safety is an interpersonal construct that can come with a great deal of both/and. For instance, we may feel safe in the thunder and lightning but not feel safe in our own home. People seeking healing ultimately need to explore what is keeping us from settling into a ventral vagal state in the present, that place from which we can respond instead of react. Enough practice with the exploration over time can bring about some true transformations in how we navigate life. In her estimation, what Holli, Katharine, and Amy share to wrap up this section indicates a shift that happens from state change (e.g., how to ground, how to keep ourselves safe enough) to trait change—experiencing the real, radical change that helps give us a deeper sense of wholeness and steadiness.

EXPRESSIVE ARTS PRACTICE: MAKING PLAYLISTS

Even if you don't see yourself as a very expressive person, chances are there is still some music you like to listen to. Listening to music and assembling it into a collection you find especially helpful or anchoring is one of the best ways to begin working with the expressive arts in your healing, particularly the art of music. As a child of the 1980s, I learned to make mixtapes at a very young age by hitting PLAY + RECORD on my tape deck as I listened to the radio. As I grew up alongside much of the technology, I transitioned to burning CDs with collections of my favorite music. Now, programs like Spotify, Apple Music, or even YouTube (you can create a free account and assemble music) make constructing playlists simpler and more accessible.

There are a variety of ways to incorporate your music and playlists into the healing process. We'll begin by inviting you to make an "After Therapy" (or other healing art) playlist. This exercise is inspired by Crystal, a former client of mine and contributor to this book, who always assured me that she was okay to drive herself home from intense therapy sessions because she *had her music*. Can you put together a collection of at least ten songs or ten musical moods (e.g., soft jazz, orchestral music, heavy metal, tribal drumming) that are rather consistent in helping you stay grounded, awake, or maybe even happy or uplifted? This is your collection and you never have to share it with anyone! If it makes you feel less self-conscious, please know that Hanson's "MMMBop" from the late 1990s is on our After Therapy playlist!

After making this core playlist, you may challenge yourself and/or your system to take it a little deeper. Consider making a second playlist along the theme of safety. Are there ten songs or ten musical moods that help you feel a little safer, especially if that sense of safety is internal? Perhaps you have a fictional character that you work with as a protector figure or resource; one of mine is Wonder Woman, complete with her gold wrist cuffs and the Lasso of Truth. Can you consult a soundtrack from one of the movies or series made for that fictional character and include them on your list?

Another variation you can use for this exercise that can be powerful, especially if you identify as having a system or working with different aspects of yourself, is to allow each member of the system or part to make their own playlist. That angsty teenage part of yours may really need to let you put together some of their own music for this one so do not censor yourselves with the genres that come up. Death metal or trap music may be appropriate. After each part gets to make their own playlist, consider comparing notes internally and composing a playlist that represents the needs of each part or aspect of self being met.

What are they noticing?

QUESTIONS TO ASK MY THERAPIST OR PSYCHIATRIST

- What is your general approach to grounding? Are you okay if I call it something else besides grounding?

- Do you have a set of specific skills that you teach your clients for grounding, or are you open to my bringing in some of my own?

- What are your feelings about incorporating Indigenous, Eastern (Asian), African, or other healing systems other than Western psychology into the healing process?

- If you don't have training to work with these types of practices, are you open to having me explore them as companions to the work we do in therapy?

- How do you handle it if I, as your client, am suddenly not feeling safe or safe enough with you? Is this something you are open to having me address?

- How do you distinguish the difference between physical and emotional safety?

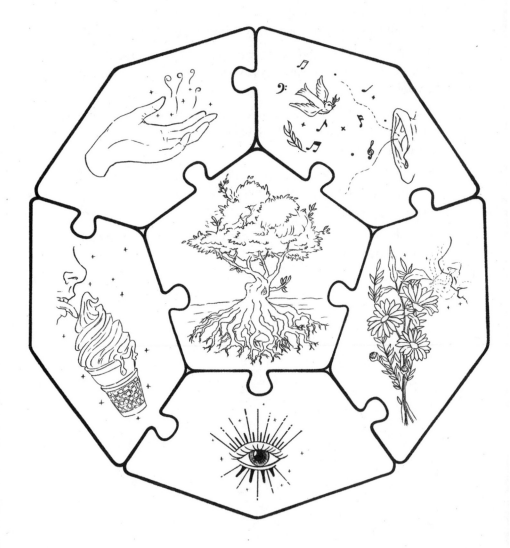

4

The Wide World of Parts and Systems: Different Styles of Dancing with Life

There are two types of beings in the universe:
those who dance and those who do not.

—DRAX THE DESTROYER, *Guardians of the Galaxy*

When I left the theater after the second installment of *Guardians of the Galaxy,* arguably the most fun franchise in the Marvel Cinematic Universe, I was weeping. Visibly and audibly weeping.

The boys I helped raise who eventually became my sons, used to the heavy displays of emotion that I can show during all kinds of movies, asked what these tears were about.

"That film was the most beautiful parts metaphor I have ever seen! I mean the first one was good for showing how a band of misfits can come together and make a family but this . . . this one, with the new characters and new dynamics! This film shows what dissociative trauma survivors with a system do to survive and even become creative in the world," I gushed.

"You're gonna have to explain that one to me," Ethan, who was twelve at the time, said with a somewhat confused look.

So as not to give too much away in case you haven't seen the movies, the original film focuses on the protagonist named Peter Quill (aka Star-Lord), a half-human, half-alien galactic bounty hunter who, interestingly enough, has a thing for dancing to mixtapes. Indeed, his human mother gave him his first mixtape just prior to her tragic death. When a bounty is later placed on Peter's head by the renegade alien who raised him, he befriends a literal cast of characters, many of whom were initially in conflict with each other, on his adventures through the universe—Rocket Raccoon, a foul-mouthed, wise-cracking genetically modified character (who doesn't believe he's a raccoon); Groot, a tree who is described as part bodyguard, part houseplant; Drax the Destroyer, a powerful warrior who thinks only in concrete terms (he would hate the amount of metaphor we're about to use in this chapter); and Gamora, a female alien—also a warrior and an assassin—raised by one of the most notorious villains in the Marvel Universe, who is attempting to atone for her past crimes and associations. They all help each other survive and defeat the evil forces that threaten to destroy them. You know, what trauma survivors have to do every day. . . .

In the second film they are joined by Mantis, an empathic bug-like crea-ture. Groot takes on a hilariously new form, and we realize that some of the characters we originally despised as villains were a lot more complicated and sympathetic than we first thought. The crew is also dealt a new challenge when we learn just how powerful the ego can be in sabotaging a sense of balance in the system, and we even meet Peter's alien birth father who gives an apt portrayal of what in systems work it might mean to align with a per-petrating part. In other words, an aspect (or part) of the victim can align very strongly with, even defend, the person who victimized them. Several of our contributors bring more nuance to this term in the chapter.

As I first mentioned in the introduction, in modern-day studies around dissociation and parts work, it is common for professionals like myself to be asked what our preferred *model* is for working with parts and systems. Is it Internal Family Systems (IFS)? Is it Theory of Structural Dissociation? Is it Jungian archetypes? For me and many of the folks I serve, learning to frame their internal system through the lens of a movie like *Guardians of the Galaxy,* or through any series of creative metaphors, is much more pow-erful. Once we can see how the aspects of ourselves relate to each other in ways that make sense to us, we can welcome these parts into greater com-munication with each other. I've also been known to lean into the *Star Wars* Universe and the original movie I bonded with at the chronological age of four, *The Wizard of Oz,* to explain my own system and other psychological concepts like the triune brain model first introduced in chapter 2. Think about it—the Cowardly Lion (who believed he lacked courage) is the brain stem, the Tin Man (who believed he lacked a heart) is the limbic system, and the Scarecrow (who believed he lacked a brain) is the neocortex. Through leaning on each other they discovered that they each had what they really needed all along, and Dorothy, our protagonist, needed all three to reconnect to her truest sense of home.

In this chapter you will read about how our contributors—those who do not have a clinically diagnosed dissociative disorder yet relate to having parts, as well as those who have a clinically diagnosed dissociative disorder—explain how their parts interplay. Some even offer insight into how they formed and/or how they were revealed. Here is an advanced insight—none of them—none of the sixty-one (even though many are knowledgeable in technical parts models) used technical model language to answer the question, "If you identify as having a parts system, how would you describe your system?" One of the contributors we've referenced several times in the book who goes by the name The Garden System literally named her system in that fashion because she used the metaphor of a garden to describe how her internal parts formed and interact with each other. I've used the *Guardians of the Galaxy* metaphor for many years now to help people understand some of how my internal system works. Yet I got chills as I wrote the opening to this chapter because many of our contributors used metaphors like galaxies and solar systems to describe their inner worlds!

Before we go into this wide world of metaphor and offer some insights and exercises inspired by the wisdom of metaphor, we will cover in a general way a definition for parts and some of the major models that are in use for parts work and addressing dissociative systems in modern therapy. In this section, we will also ask you to consider how working with parts and aspects of self predates people like Richard Schwartz and Carl Jung. This exploration will begin with an examination of some Indigenous wisdom.

Introducing Parts and Exploring Various Models for Parts Work

Adam O'Brien, whom we've met several times throughout the book, believes there are two types of people in the world—not necessarily those who dance and those who don't. To Adam, everyone has a system, there are just people who realize that they do, and people who are not yet aware of theirs. Recall Roger Vielle's wisdom offered in the introductory chapter, informed by decades of his own recovery and steeping in Blackfeet tradition—"We are all our own universe within a universe." Roger's teaching is an elegant way of saying there are many components that can make up who we are. For people with unhealed trauma, those components might become more separated and distinct, phenomena that our contributors will share about throughout the chapter.

Parts is a general term used in the psychological and helping professions that can refer to many different things. I see it as the most generic term possible that can be used to describe aspects, sides, or facets of self that do not necessarily represent the presence of another ego state. Some people even conceptualize their parts as the various roles they occupy in life, for instance: mother, teacher, friend, client, bowler, social justice advocate, etc. In the modern-day helping professions, many models for *parts work* address the idea that all human beings have parts. *Ego states* is another term relevant to this discussion. A psychoanalytic term based in Freud's concept of *ego* (derived from the Latin word for "I"), ego states generally refer to aspects of the client's personality based in unresolved material (e.g., the frightened child). Although these ego states can feel separate and distinct, they do not necessarily contain the degree of fragmentation that would be required for a part to be considered a dissociative alter.

In the dissociation scholarship, *alter* has been adapted from *alter ego* to reference an alternate or changed self that is a separate and distinct personality. Popular culture is once again full of *alter ego* examples in superheroes and villains alike, and these switches—some of which are more subtle and some of which are more pronounced—can add richness and depth to a narrative. Many people with DID refer to their other self or collection of other selves as alters based on this traditional conceptualization of the term. *Introject* parts, based on a term from Gestalt therapy, can refer to parts that are intruding with the process of the core self or the entire system, and sometimes seem to align with a perpetrator or an abusive figure.

There can be many terms to keep straight when you are first learning about dissociation and DID. Kathleen, a former preschool teacher with DID whom we met in the previous chapter reflects, "All of the terminology can sound Greek and foreign when you are first diagnosed. Once you wade through it, it makes sense." Recognizing that this terminology can indeed feel overwhelming, we remind you that there is a glossary of terms at the beginning of the book that can help you with the wading. That glossary may come in extra handy during this chapter. As a personal aside, I/we would like to say that in your healing process, whether you identify as having DID or some other issue, the terminology you choose is completely up to you. Both Dr. Jamie and Jamie dislike the terms *alters* and *introjects*—we see them both as outdated and feel that leaning into the language of *parts* is most neutral and least stigmatizing, whether you're discussing DID or another diagnosis. Yet Kathleen and Sandra Johnson are two contributors who don't like the word *parts*. Kathleen says, "Parts make me sound like a car. I prefer to call the members of my system *defenders*." Sandra simply prefers the term *selves*. The key to trauma-informing anything is that you can always modify the language and if you are working with a professional, it's important that they understand that language may very much matter to you.

Indigenous and Pre-Jungian Perspectives

In listening to some of our Indigenous contributors and practitioners of Shamanic and Celtic healing arts, we obtain further insight into just how limiting the perspectives of Western psychology can be. For Susan Pease Banitt, a clinical social worker trained at a hospital within the Harvard Medical School system—yet more open to the healing traditions of her Celtic origins and other Indigenous traditions, Western perspectives are about shrinking a person's reality. She goes on to say, "I don't like the word *system*, it's too mechanical. I prefer the word *multidimensional*."

For Jasa Johnson, Western models in general are too pathologizing and do not allow for human beings to live in a state of wholeness. In the traditions of Shamanism in which Jasa trained, everything speaks, you just have to give yourself a chance to listen to it. In modern therapy-speak, Jasa translates this to, "Every part is valid, every part has a voice . . . and your parts will never lie to you." When Jasa hears Western psychological teaching on dissociation, these resonate for her as the concept of *soul loss,* or the splitting off of aspects of self. According to Jasa, this split happens because the psyche seeks to protect you in the wake of any kind of trauma or wound, even the things that may not seem so big on the surface. Jasa describes how this informs the approach she takes to helping others on their healing journey:

> Someone has to go into the void to retrieve those parts and convince them to come back. They won't come back if they can't be assured that they will be safe. The Shaman dialogues with the part on their person's behalf. Sometimes it's not appropriate for the parts to come back. Sometimes it's better that it stays in the void, but you can do a release, thanking the part for the teaching that it brought. The decision to "re-integrate" or rejoin is totally up to those parts.

Although Julian Jaramillo, the Ecuadorian Shaman trained and ordained in the traditions of the Chocó people, is well steeped in the language of parts and Jungian archetypes through his own psychological training, to his Chocó teacher there is no conception of parts. To his teacher and in traditional wisdom, mythology *is* reality. So if an individual seeking healing is from a certain place, they would be well-steeped in the stories and traditions of that place, and the gifted healer works with them to align and relate to those stories so a person could connect to their personal meaning in that story. For example, in the mythology of his Shaman's village the *washu,* or monkey that is an endangered species, often shows up in his visions as choking the neck of a person who is suicidal, especially if the afflicted person lost a child. In that tradition the *washu* is believed to hunt babies to unite them with the path of the Great Mother, or death. So if his Shaman sees the monkey choking someone who is depressed or suicidal in one of his visions, he has to work with removing the spirit of that monkey so that the person's shadow can be cleansed.

Needless to say, it is not a stretch for Julian to see the wisdom of a person working with their preferred metaphors and myths, even if they are Marvel movies, to help them understand themselves and what keeps them from connecting with wholeness. My journey over the past several years has taught me that while *parts work* is being hailed as an invention of Western psychology that has come into a light of new understanding with models like IFS gaining popularity; working with parts, aspects, or dimensions of self is nothing new. If you can appreciate mythology and belief systems, especially on a global perspective, this idea will resonate.

When I deepened into my yoga study several years ago, I became interested in learning about the mythologies of India. Growing up as a kid in a Catholic school in the midwestern United States, I learned that Hinduism is a polytheistic religion, or a religion of many gods. This is false. In Hindu mythology, there is One supreme God, but God manifests in over 300 million ways. And the gods we hear about such as Krishna, Radha, Sita, Ram, Ganesh, and Hanuman are the stories of how Divine presence expresses themselves in the world. And once you learn more about the stories and how the expressions interplay, a treasure trove of connections to the human experience emerges.

My favorite story involves the monkey god Hanuman, which originally appeared in a Sanskrit epic called the *Ramayana.* In Hindu mythology, female and male deities are usually referenced together, symbolizing the sacred unity between energy (feminine) and consciousness (masculine). Once, the demon Ravan (who represents the ego) lured and captured Sita to exploit her for his own benefit. Ram called upon his devoted servant, the beloved monkey Hanuman, who represents the heart, the breath, and the ability to adapt or shapeshift to any situation depending on how he is needed. As a monkey, he is also seen as a bridge between the human and animal worlds. Hanuman called upon the forces of his entire monkey army and they found Sita at the southern tip of India, rescuing her so she could be reunited with her beloved. Hanuman's role in this story represents the power of the breath to reunite energy and consciousness. In this powerful fusion of energy and consciousness joined by the breath, order is restored and we are deeply healed.

Another fabulous insight that I received from the Hindu tradition came from a driver of mine in India named Sonu. As a man of great devotion yet without any special theological training, he told me, "Pray to Ganesh first." Ganesh is the elephant god known as the remover of obstacles. Sonu continued, "You need the obstacles to be removed for anything else to happen, right? So pray to Ganesh first." I've put this teaching to work so many times for myself in asking, "What part or aspect of me is standing in the way of my showing up how I want to be in the world? And can Ganesh be a resource for that part to help clear the obstacle away?"

One of the reasons we can study any mythology is to notice what the characters reveal about ourselves and how we may relate to the world. As another teacher of mine in these traditions shared with me when I told him of my dissociative disorder diagnosis, "You know, some views of the Hindu canon teach that a *demon* is a part that just tries to make itself the whole thing, acting out so to speak, and not work with the totality." Hearing this teaching was another example of that proverbial lightning of recognition shooting through my veins. Even the metaphor of *demon* as it gets used in Western psychology contexts can suggest that demons are bad and need to be slain. Yet in Hindu mythology and some schools of Buddhism (namely Tibetan Buddhism), the demons need to be addressed, heard, or even fed and nourished.[5] Then natural healing can occur.

If these examples from Hindu mythology and Buddhist tradition feel like too much of a stretch for you because of where you are coming from spiritually or religiously, I encourage you to bring up your own religious tradition. What might the saints or sacred figures and their stories teach you about your relationship to the world? Is there a sacred figure you connect with more strongly than others? Is there one who represents parts or aspects of yourself that have long remained in shadow? And if you are not spiritual or religious at all, keep using other mythologies that may appeal to you, which can include fictional works like the Marvel, Disney, or *Star Wars* universes . . . or really anything your heart desires.

Jungian Archetypes

Carl Jung (1875–1961), the Swiss psychiatrist considered one of the fathers of psychoanalysis and depth psychology, believed in the concept of the *collective unconscious.* The collective unconscious is that unconscious mind that contains instincts and what Jung called archetypes. In a more current review of Carl Jung and his legacy, John O'Brien summarized, "Archetypes are universal organizing themes or patterns that appear regardless of space, time, or person. Appearing in all existential realms and at all levels of systematic recursion, they are organized as themes in the *unus mundus* [one world], which Jung . . . described as 'the potential world outside of time,' and are detectable through synchronicities."[6]

The main archetypal frameworks that Jung taught can be roughly categorized as such:

ARCHETYPAL EVENTS

- birth
- death
- separation from parents
- initiation
- marriage
- the union of opposites

ARCHETYPAL FIGURES

- great mother (can exist opposite to the bad mother)
- father (can exist opposite to the bad father)
- child
- devil
- god
- wise old man
- wise old woman
- the trickster

- the hero
- the shapeshifter

ARCHETYPAL MOTIFS

- the apocalypse
- the deluge
- creation

Jung also wrote of other concepts that weave into the collective unconscious of the human experience: the *self* (unity of personality as a whole and
the wide range of our psychic phenomena), the *shadow* (sometimes seen as
the dark side or the aspects we've not yet examined; may run counter to our
values), and the *anima/animus* (sexual energies). Jung acknowledged that this
list is not exhaustive, as archetypes and their combinations are constantly
revealing themselves. If you are a fan of mythologies and cinematic universes
(like Marvel, *Star Wars, Harry Potter, Lord of the Rings,* etc.), perhaps notice
which archetypes that appear here may correspond with some of your favorite characters. As an example, Yoda in the *Star Wars* Universe can be described
as a blend between the wise old man and the Trickster. Shapeshifters show up
frequently in mythologies, and this archetype is one that many people with
dissociative experiences of life can relate to.

Naturally, the work of Carl Jung, as with many early leaders in modern
psychology, has come under criticism for not being sufficiently grounded in
science and not sufficiently feminist. In my view, there is always room for a
feminist update of traditional concepts that may carry some value, and archetypes are no exception. And as you can imagine, many in the modern era are
put off by the obvious mystical and metaphysical quality of Jung's beliefs and
writings. Yet his embrace of something larger than the physical body and
mind is something we are calling for in this book and in a more enlightened
approach to working with dissociation and parts. Julian Jaramillo, a student
of depth psychology in his life as a trained psychologist, believes there are
many parallels between what his Shamanic elder taught him and what Jung
developed. And his elder never read a word of Jung.

In my healing journey, for several years I worked with an expressive arts
therapist trained in Jungian archetypes and I found the work very valuable
in helping me identify how some of the needs and desires of my parts were
indeed buried in the shadows. Sinking into the archetype of the shapeshifter
as a way to frame my dissociative mind proved to be nonpathologizing and

helpful to my process, allowing me to frame so many of my experiences and how I see the world as gifts. I found these revelations helped enhance the work that I was doing in other therapeutic models and helped give me another frame for understanding parts.

Ego State Therapy

An early model for working with parts that remains in use is ego state therapy, which originates in the psychodynamic tradition as well. Originally developed by John and Helen Watkins, ego state therapy posits that distinct and rigid ego state development (as we may see in DID) is not the norm, yet most every individual's personality contains various parts or states that may need to be addressed. The "inner child" is a classic example of such a part or state used in ego state therapy, and the "control freak" may be another.[7] Many psychotherapeutic approaches and techniques can be used to achieve a sense of internal harmony, or diplomacy, within a person's system of parts. Many overlaps with Jungian archetypes appear in this system of working with parts, roles, and aspects of self.

Fraser's Table

Many trauma-focused therapists find that Fraser's Table is a solid place to begin the concept of *parts* or *system mapping* with their clients. If you are working with a trauma-focused therapist to address dissociation, they may have you try this exercise. Psychiatrist George Fraser, an advocate who worked to spread recognition of DID, believed that a person with dissociative parts could get to know their system and how the various parts interact with each other. His original article led to the popularization of the "conference table" metaphor for people being able to map out their parts and how they interact. Fraser offered a variety of other metaphorical possibilities for this mapping, with an emphasis that the table metaphor is only one part of his larger technique.[8]

In the original article from 1991, Fraser presents the following approaches:

- Relaxation Imagery: refers to using guided imagery as preparation and resourcing.

- Dissociative Table Imagery: credited as Gestalt in nature, Fraser sees this as the most important component of the exercise, using the principle of imagery for a client to begin seeing their internal system take seats around a table. He also discusses some modifications if tables feel unsafe.

- The Spotlight Technique: shines a spotlight on the alter (or part) who is directly speaking to the therapist. Modifications are available if the light feels unsafe.

- The Middleman Technique: establishes a system of communication between the alters (or parts) where one can speak on behalf of several others. In this technique and in the article generally he addresses the concept of *co-consciousness,* referring to two or more parts/alters sharing consciousness at the same time (i.e., not blacking out, "going away," etc.).

- The Screen Technique: a distancing technique where distressing memories can be viewed as if they are on a screen in the same room as the table.

- The Search for the Center Ego State (Inner Self Helper): reveals what may sometimes be referred to as the "core self" of the presenting self that has the strongest overview/sense of the entire system. Controversy exists over whether it's necessary for some dissociative systems to even have a Center Ego State, as many (including The Garden System in this book) report not having one.

- Memory Projection Technique: furthers communication between the various alters/parts and their memories, using the various parts to bring in resources as other states may work to process or heal other memories on the screen.

- Transformation Stage Technique: transforms a person's relationship to the memory and how they see themselves in the memory in terms of time, space, and age.

The final approach in Fraser's article addresses the issue of fusion or integration, a strong area of potential controversy for those diagnosed with or identifying as DID. Many individuals with DID strongly resist or oppose a psychiatrist or any other provider's insistence that they *integrate* the various aspects of their personality into a cohesive whole. This process can feel disrespectful to the members of a system, and if you are reading this passage and have ever felt triggered at the suggestion that you need to integrate, you are not alone. In the following section where contributors speak to how their systems operate, you will read many insights around whether the word and concept of *integration* works (for two of our contributors it does), or whether other ways of looking at healing (e.g., cohesion, unity, community, diplomacy) are a better fit.

Theory of Structural Dissociation

Fraser's Table is arguably one of the most popular approaches in the first wave of dissociation studies following the formal introduction of dissociative disorders into DSM-III in 1980, and the Theory of Structural Dissociation is the other major player. Developed by Onno van der Hart, Ellert Nijenhuis, and Kathy Steele, the theory is widely embraced by trauma-focused therapists because many consider it nonpathologizing, asserting that we are all born with a fragmented or dissociative mind. This fragmentation is how infants get their various needs met in the absence of speech, language, or a more developed neocortex. The presence of healthy development allows for a natural integration of the personality structure. Yet in the presence of unhealed trauma, disorganized attachment, or developmental distress, a natural separation is bound to remain.[9]

The two main terms used in the Theory of Structural Dissociation are *apparently normal personality (ANP)*, which is similar to Fraser's idea of the Center Ego State, and *emotional part of the personality (EP)*. Emotional parts remain to protect or to meet a need, and some systems contain a more complicated interconnection of EPs and ANPs than others. The model uses the terms *primary structural dissociation* (which we are more likely to see in PTSD and other trauma-related disorders), *secondary dissociation* (indicative of personality disorders, dissociative disorders other than DID, and complex PTSD or developmental trauma) and *tertiary dissociation* (classically presented as DID).

The Theory of Structural Dissociation, like every model presented in this section, has garnered criticism. Dr. Colin Ross offered a modification to the theory. He posits that emotional personalities (EPs) do not have to be separate entities in and of themselves, rather, they can hold a fragment or experience like a thought, feeling, memory, or sensation. This modification may be easier for clients struggling with addiction as dissociation to consider. In this modification to the model, Ross expands on Pierre Janet's ideas that many disorders can be viewed through the lens of dissociation.[10]

In our view, the Theory of Structural Dissociation was a step in the right direction yet remains incomplete in and of itself. Ross's updates give greater permission to modify, which is essential for any care to be more trauma- and dissociation-informed. I remember the first time I heard someone present on the Theory of Structural Dissociation and use these *ANP/EP* terms at a conference, my head completely shut down. Many of us with a dissociative experience of life are displeased with the adjective *normal* to describe the core self or presenting adult (ANP). For many folks struggling with dissociation, this label has historically felt insulting although many proponents of the Theory of Structural Dissociation are becoming increasingly open to modifications in language around the theory's terminology.

Internal Family Systems

For many trauma-focused professionals, the term *Internal Family Systems (IFS)*, developed by Richard Schwartz, is even less pathologizing and more user-friendly than the Theory of Structural Dissociation. There are countless training courses on IFS and on blending IFS with other models of therapy like EMDR Therapy. At the time of this writing IFS is the model I am asked about most frequently, and it seems like the most popular current model for working with parts. Even Schwartz's most recent book, *No Bad Parts: Healing Trauma and Restoring Wholeness with the Internal Family Systems Model* features a foreword from popular musician Alanis Morisette.

A major contention of IFS is that the core of a person is the *Self,* which is inherently whole and undamaged.[11] This teaching is quite aligned with what yoga philosophy teaches about the Self. The three major types of parts that form to protect the core Self are *exiles* (created by trauma, generally seen as the parts we are hesitant to look at or examine), *managers* (created to protect the Self from the exiles), and *firefighters* (created to put out strong emotions and keep the exiles contained). In the example of substance use disorders, addictive or other acting-out behavior is a function of the firefighting parts, and the manager parts may stand in the way of a person and their system addressing what they need to in order to heal (the exiles).

The IFS approach can make good sense to most of my clients when giving them an explanation of what parts are and how they interact with each other. The idea that we are already built to be whole is fundamentally very empowering. The IFS movement is also accelerating the conversation that we all have parts and that all of our parts are to be honored, which is an idea that I fundamentally believe and highlight as a major truth in this book. For myself and several of my professional collaborators, while we can see the value of IFS popularity in carrying this message, we also have concerns that the needs and complexities of people with DID and other dissociative disorders run the risk of being erased or even disparaged. Several on my team were very upset to read, in a new book on IFS by Dr. Frank Anderson (which was endorsed by Bessel van der Kolk and featured a foreword by Richard Schwartz), how people with DID were portrayed. One phrase, calling people with DID "masters of deception" struck them as highly problematic.[12] Another book seeking to mainstream parts work, James Fadiman and Jordan Gruber's *Your Symphony of Selves: Discover and Understand More of Who We Are,* does have some helpful content that I cited in chapter I. Yet the overall tone of that book is rather discouraging because it seeks to encourage a *dissociation* between more "normal" parts understanding in the general population and people with dissociative diagnoses.

Metaphors and Meaning: The Wisdom of Our Contributors

As you read on in this section, listening to our contributors who speak about their systems and inner worlds; you will likely see more similarities than differences—regardless of diagnosis—on how systems develop, form, and exist in the world. We do not expect all of these metaphors and descriptions to resonate for you, yet we urge you to pay attention to those that do. You are also encouraged to notice that for people with dissociative disorders, having their systems understood, respected, and not put into any kind of neatly boxed-in model can be imperative to their thriving in the world. For organizational purposes, we've first elected to feature contributors who do not report a dissociative disorder diagnosis of any kind, but do relate to having parts or even a system. Next, we will explore the voices of people with OSDD or other dissociative disorders that do not meet full criteria for DID, and then move to our contributors who report a DID diagnosis. As a special section, we will then feature the experiences of our two contributors (one with DID and one with dissociative features as a result of complex trauma) who now identify as being integrated.

Contributors with an Identified System and No Clear Dissociative Disorder Diagnosis

My collaborator Adam O'Brien provided us with perhaps our favorite metaphor we've heard since setting out on this work. Adam's description gives us a nature-based metaphor that can help us understand how we can all have parts, yet for some of us the definition of those parts may be more pronounced. When a tree is cut down, the stump leaves behind a series of rings or grooves that approximate how long the tree has lived, with one circular groove representing one year. Adam reflects that while each ring (i.e., year, part) is relevant to the structure of the tree, some grooves are a little more noticeable, depending on what happened during that year. If the rings are skinny, conditions were likely more drought-like in that year. In the healthy years with good water, the grooves are more pronounced. In Adam's view, our inner architecture may metaphorically look like those rings of a tree, with each year of our lives able to reveal more about the conditions of our lives and internal world at that time.

Holli Ellis sees her parts as different photographs that make up an album, which is helpful to her as someone who is very visual. There are four distinct parts that she identifies: one that feels most like her authentic self, and three others that she can recall from different parts of her life. Her seven-year-old part is the most likely to get activated. Says Holli, "If she shows up, I must be doing *this*..." and then she knows she needs to attend to that part very gently.

Thomas Zimmerman has a system that he sees as existing at a small table, even though they are not so differentiated. The young boy part, who is somewhere between the ages of seven and thirteen, comes up a lot in the context of anger. Other parts are connected to his trauma from being bullied in middle school and have the potential to completely freeze him. He also names an analytical or "postmodern" part that initially served a significant role in helping him "make sense of the rubble." Yet Thomas also reflects, "That identity makes you live your life on the territory of a postage stamp."

Danyale Weems also does not see herself as disintegrated or split. Yet when she does need to interact with her parts and what they represent (e.g., pleasure), she finds the metaphor of the living room as the core of a house to be useful. The living room is her core self, and when she notices that parts are jumping into the living room too much, she needs to pay attention to them.

Crystal is one of our contributors who uses a galaxy metaphor to help her understand herself. She says that she can internalize it as such, although it's not something she necessarily feels and sees. Crystal identifies separate and distinct parts within this galaxy—an inner child (whom she can hate), an angry part (whom her partner has pointed out), and a separating part that formed when her chronic illness took away her ability to ride horses competitively, which until that point had been her best coping skill.

The following contributors do not present metaphors to describe their internal system, yet they do offer some valuable reflections on how their systems are composed and interact. Fiona identifies five parts in their system, with one specifically representing their gender dysphoria. At the time when Fiona started working on themselves, they saw them as causing problems. Now that they have worked on their parts for years and years, there is much harmony and cooperation in the system. Fiona reflects, "The angry part (seven) can sometimes tell me to set myself on fire. Now I can hear that and know that something got in and I can ask that part to determine what someone did to cross a boundary." Kylie says, "I'm still working to identify my parts. There is definitely a younger child, a younger teenager, and some critics that remind me of females I grew up with."

Blaise identifies approximately six parts: anger (a gorilla in a cage, shaking, always trying to get out), the jealous guy (his age can fluctuate), the kid (about age eight, prone to abandonment), the jokester (creates chaos and tries to make everyone happy), and the skeptical guy. His sixth part represents his depression; he knows it's there but doesn't want to put a name to it, saying, "It's like one of those friends with benefits that wants to keep coming in, it's always there." Erin calls her system *parts* even though she doesn't feel "super fragmented." She identifies Eight (carefree and enjoyable, aligned with her authentic self), Penny (about twelve years old, a "fake" protector), Sixteen (the moody adolescent part who cut herself), and Baby Therapist, whom she describes as "When Sixteen grew up and had some cognitive behavioral therapy."

Rebecca (age forty-four at the time of our interview) states that she does not have her parts named but that they are "a part of her"—one is her ten-year-old self (when molestation happened) and the other is twenty-seven years old (when she experienced a major medical trauma). Malika categorizes her parts more as "natural versus unnatural" or "being in my essence and effortless ... or not." sunnEe hope uses an archetypal system that she learned from teacher Caroline Myss to help her organize her parts: a young part, an angry teenager, a wise old crone, an addict. She says, "They get along pretty well these days, they all have good intentions, even the most seemingly harmful ones." Rachael says that she does not see herself as having a very identified system as she sees in many of her clients, yet when her little part shows up (who is about eight), "I need to engage and interact with her." Paula S. sees her parts as "all me," yet she will shift into different emotional states as they are needed and those states will have different levels of maturity: therapist/professional, hurt/deprived, "Bronx Paula" (can scare anyone and would "love to be an assassin"), child/carefree, nasty/bratty teenager, the fawn part.

Elizabeth Davis identifies a series of survival-focused parts that she didn't come to work on until her mid-forties, largely inspired by her own IFS training. She identifies parts that are four, five, and seven; a part that is a dog; and a managing part "that has become softer over the years." Tada Hozumi identifies Japanese Tada, street culture Tada, femme parts, and male parts, reflecting, "Dance is one of the ways that you can combine the parts together."

Jackson identifies strongly as having a "Sacred Clown" part from certain Native American traditions: "the one who is always smiling and dancing through life, living a message of hope." He also connects with Asu Allegra from African mythology as his current protector part; Asu Allegra is "the character who can turn anything upside down." He sees these parts as being healthier replacements for his prior protector stance of "ghetto intellectual," trying to show everyone how smart he is. In the end, he realized how much this part alienated people. Chuck Bernsohn has been much more aware of their protector parts of late, and current work has centered on integrating self-love into parts work. While Chuck identifies as having a wisest, oldest self, their younger parts have "been such a joy to meet." Chuck continues, "The interaction between them has only happened in the container of spiritual work."

Contributors with an Identified System and a Dissociative Disorder Diagnosis Other than DID

Danielle is a practicing therapist in long-term recovery from an opioid use disorder who was only ever diagnosed by someone else with PTSD, yet identifies highly with the OSDD descriptors. She came to know and understand her system first through taking an expressive arts–based course I teach on understanding dissociation. Although she trained in EMDR Therapy with my program, she worked with a separate and distinct therapist who helped her more fully understand her system. Danielle connects very strongly with the Russian nesting doll as a metaphor (the wooden doll where you open an outer layer, and then smaller inner layers of the same doll continue to be revealed). Danielle has purchased nesting dolls with a variety of outer shells—Wonder Woman (representing a protector part and Superhero Mom), a princess, other superheroes, more traditional dolls—to help her set up and understand her parts map. As it stands, there are eleven distinct dolls (with their layers) placed on a horizontally oriented map. Working in the various directions with her mapping helps her honor the complexity.

In general, Danielle sees her ANP as a woman in recovery, seeking growth, presence, and connection. Yet there are a number of other parts and variations that can come out and show up in different forms and at different times. Danielle generally categorizes these other parts as Inner Child, Essence, Addiction, Lost Girl, Dissociative Parts, Guilt/Shame, Protector Parts, Wife, and Inner Wisdom. Thus, having the multiple planes to express her system (the horizontal map and the multilayered dolls who stand vertically) makes the most sense to her.

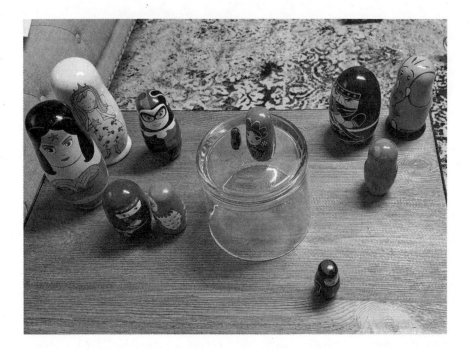

A.J., who is diagnosed with OSDD, describes a very intricate understanding of her system that she can loosely see existing visually as a Venn diagram. She is in her late twenties, and exists in an overlap between A (the "common thread; the body's story is her story") and Jane (developed in her mid-twenties, with very strong "Mary Poppins" energy, "the literal personification of executive function"). Her other parts are Kiddo (age six, the "soft heart" at the center of their system); Cassidy (late teens, "unbridled teenage fangirl enthusiasm; her energy feels like pop rocks in my body"); and Mia (late twenties, "quiet, hasn't shown herself much yet; she feels like a rich bass line"). A.J. sees herself as having a very cohesive relationship with her system. She observes that she and Jane "co-front" a great deal, and approach the demands of graduate school "like a team."

Andrea, who shared about her experiences with a Derealization diagnosis in chapter 1, initially conceptualized her system as a conference table, yet that's evolved to referring to them as a "crew." As a lover of nature, which is imperative for helping her and the crew stay grounded, Andrea sees them as living in a teepee in the woods along a river. She sees this as a symbolic protection against everything else in the world. The crew contains a strong four-year-old part (who has an opinion about everything), and other parts that are conscious of any situations involving stress. For instance, these parts can become very activated when going to the dentist, and Andrea needs to prep them with things to do before going in.

One of our anonymous contributors identifies a system of parts with different functions, and "needing to work with them to stay grounded and managing them is an important part of my daily routine." There are two "abandonment" parts (one is a baby, another is age five) that show up as sensations in her body. There is an eighteen-year-old part, a pain part (which announces that "something is up"), an anger part, another young part that retreats under a table, and an intense work part. Alicia Hann sees her parts as "all me, but at different ages." There is a young, shy child (about the age she was when a major trauma took place); a teenage part that represents the eating disorder, ballet, and self-hatred; and a college-age part connected to a lot of shame. She says, "For the most part they are willing to have a conversation, but it may depend on the topic."

Contributors with an Identified System and Dissociative Identity Disorder (DID)

Two of our contributors with DID make use of the solar system metaphor. Melissa Parker, a therapist with DID in her late forties, says that the solar system represents that "we are all of these things, all in our place." For the longest time she was convinced that she was the person and she had a lot of parts. Yet she's come to realize through her healing that "We are complete in ourselves. We are not just our parts. Even on our own, we would be complete people." Melissa, who believes that there are major flaws with the Theory of Structural Dissociation covered earlier in this chapter, mostly rejects it because it is monolithic and not written by "people like us." She further comments, "I see new parts as growth, not damage. We are people and not just parts."

Amy Brickler, the therapist with DID whom we met in chapter 2 as she discussed her congenital brain trauma, said that her system mates revealed themselves to her following a mental health episode in adulthood that involved her self-injury. Amy explains, "As clearly as I'm seeing you right now a little girl appeared before me and told me her name and why she was here—and that in the next days I would be meeting three others. And she was very clear about who we could trust to tell about this, because other people wouldn't understand." Through time and her healing journey, she's come to view her system mates, who she says do not switch very much, as a solar system. The more system mates that revealed themselves, the more natural it became to group them on a planetary map.

In her healing, Amy eventually came to draw her core self as the sun in the center of her solar system. She indicates that at first her system mates seemed annoyed by this, thinking that she was "over them." Yet Amy communicated, "I'm not over you. I just wasn't feeling like I was a part of you. So I made myself the sun." While she said it initially felt strange to plant that flag of the sun in her map of the solar system, which also uses the name "The Souls," after their dialogue she then heard the message, "You are a part of The Souls."

A question often arises about whether people with DID identify with having a core self or whether they are purely a system. Amy's description is one example of how the relationship can play out metaphorically. While most of the DID contributors to the *Dissociation Made Simple* project identify as having a core self and other more distinguished parts, The Garden System, as mentioned previously, sees themselves as a pure system without a defined core. One of the youngest parts, Daisy, named them The Garden System because she loves the visual of a garden and wanted them to be a garden. The Garden System says they really don't know any other way to be in the world, even though they use their legal name to work in their profession as a financial advisor.

They reflect, "We are lonely, but never alone."

The Garden System reports that they switch a lot, needing to schedule a lot of breaks to manage that energy. Prior to their DID diagnosis, they didn't really understand what was happening with them. Even though they had a sense of some of their names, they had no clue about multiplicity until they received the diagnosis. The Garden System recalls, "When we were little we tried to go by other names and ask people to use them, but we got in trouble for that."

A question (and controversy) that surfaces around DID is whether people with DID recognize their parts along the way, or whether work with therapists puts them there. To be honest, sometimes I've even questioned that myself in my own healing journey. And then I remember the pieces of behavioral evidence, like being told I was beaned in the head with a fastball during elementary school, and I clearly see how my system formed. The Garden System remembers this strong sense of wanting to be called names other than her birth name. For Amy Wagner, who sees her twenty-six-part system as a "pretty robust system of warriors," as a kid she never had a thought that anything was developing; she just "was."

Amy, who does use an *I* pronoun and identifies as Amy, says that when she was little and surviving abuse, her system was just there—it was her comfort, her security, her safety, her companionship, her play, her wonder, her curiosity, and her survival. She thought that everyone heard voices in their head! Amy is very clear to note that her therapist did not introduce her parts. Rather, their conversations started with the rather organic "Part of me wants to yell, part of me wants to cry" in response to her therapist's questions, and from there the understanding emerged.

Jaime Pollack doesn't get caught up on the terminology, saying, "I don't care what you call them." Metaphors that she can use include a *team* of all her ego states working together as one giant ego state at this point. She also uses the metaphor of different departments that work for the same company. She explains, "It took a while to keep the departments from one-upping each other. Initially one didn't trust the other to complete the job the way it should have been completed. It took a lot of therapy and a lot of respect building to get to a place where everyone is now pretty good for each other."

Katarina Lundgren, who identifies as having approximately two hundred parts—some are purely fragments, and about twenty-five are truly active. She thinks there is some core of her, but not a specific "one of us." She uses the metaphor of hidden treasure to describe this phenomenon. At times she can see them existing as different color-coded families: blue, green, red, black, brown, yellow/shiny. She says that some of them are very free-floating, for instance, "I have a ten-year-old part with eight of their own protectors."

Christy Dunn, a therapist with DID, uses the language of camps to describe her system. She explained that there are two different, major "camps"—the abandonment parts (mostly oriented toward attachment issues and needing to attain attachment) and the powerless parts. The militaristic tone of camps feels appropriate because they often have competing goals. Christy has identified about seven abandonment parts and twelve powerless parts (one of whom is a perpetrator part). In speaking to the perpetrator part, a phenomenon in DID work that can be hard for people and their systems to grasp, Christy said that the part initially represented the primary rapist involved in her rape at age twenty-two. In her personal therapy, it came forward that this part carries the shame and the responsibility that can be a defense against some of the vulnerability and powerlessness. As they did more processing, the part came to look more like her instead of him, helping her to address some of her own trauma reenactments around sex. Christy has also identified a couple of system-related parts that help her get through life: the gatekeeper or stage manager (who can turn things hazy), the autopilot part (keeps her moving on default), and the "Robot Dory" part who operates with the wisdom of "just keep swimming, just keep swimming," inspired by the character Dory in the film *Finding Nemo*.

Megan, the paramedic we first met in chapter 2, sees her body as the "shell," and all of her approximately eight parts live inside. She has two little child parts, a middle-aged man and woman who serve as gatekeepers, a young girl, a young boy, very angry parts, a professional part, and one tied to a relationship she was in. Continuing the explanation of the shell, "If the turtle gets scared, it clams up and then can come back out as a different part." Although she didn't develop awareness of her parts until later in life, she's learned that developing internal communication with her parts has been key. This theme of learning to communicate with the system in a way that works for the system and how it relates to the world is resonant throughout the interviews with our DID contributors.

Here are some perspectives from contributors with DID that are not necessarily metaphorical in nature, yet very insightful. Alexis has eleven parts that range in age from four to adulthood. Three of her smaller parts are "buddies" with some of the older ones, and they watch out for each other. Each of her parts has their own safe space inside of her head. She explains, "One has a castle guarded by a dragon named Chauncey, and another has a tent in the woods guarded by two bears, Benjamin and Elliott." In her understanding, all of her parts were there in the beginning and some of them stopped aging when the different traumas happened and they stopped developing at that age. Now that she's done some hard therapeutic work, she is piecing more things together.

Heather (LS) Scarboro+ says, "It's like a family. This is our internal family system. We never had a system name picked out although we identified with the willow tree early on and if we had to pick a system name, it would be something like The Willow Collective." Heather (LS+) explains that everybody has a say and (for the most part now) everyone behaves, although after some problematic behavior emerged (e.g., one part running up $15,000 of credit card debt in a day) the system had to meet to establish verbal and often written contracts. Their developing rule as a system is, "We're all stuck in this body, so what do we need?"

Sandra Johnson, who at the chronological age of sixty-six is one of our oldest contributors, sees most of her parts as pretty well-integrated except for Angel, her youngest part. She prefers the word *selves* instead of *parts* but will use *parts* because people relate to it. She also dislikes the word *system*. For her, being like this is just who she is. Kathleen, the other contributor who does not like the word *parts*, says that her *defenders* live within her as in rooms of a house. Sometimes it feels as if they are living in a separate and distinct house nearby. Kathleen says that during the horrific abuse she experienced, she was there but she wasn't there; the defenders were there to help her through it. Through therapy she's gotten to know her defenders better and they communicate more effectively; the defenders all refer to her as "Big K."

Katharine, who identifies as having a core self yet has always felt a sense of parts within her, uses her own version of Fraser's Table to help her make sense of her system—which contains parts that are four, six, eleven, and fifteen. She also identifies "The Voice," who is a perpetrator-identifying part. "The Voice" scares the rest of the system, is male in nature, and dwells on topics around religion and shame. Over time and through her own work he has shifted and with her healing he doesn't feel so much like he needs to take over. For Katharine it's about noticing and naming the signals and triggers that may cause him to emerge. "It's important that I don't run and hide from him anymore; I try to communicate with him. I validate that he protected me from something at some point and has helped me in some way, even if I'm not fully aware how. The fact that I don't fight with him as much keeps him from taking over."

Cheryl describes her ten-to-twelve-part system as working together in a benevolent relationship. As she noted in chapter 1, "It's like having a family in your head ... and sometimes you don't get along with your family." Cheryl reflects that she knows the parts are "all her," but sometimes it doesn't feel that way. Sarah Smith, who is in her sixties chronologically, is still on a journey of really beginning to identify her system, saying, "I am aware of some parts more than others. I have a five-year-old part that is mischievous and a troublemaker. I recently became aware of an angry part that's around age thirteen to fourteen that I'm afraid to look at. But if I don't acknowledge it, it will be there anyway...." And John Fugett, who received his OSDD diagnosis about a year before being interviewed, says that "how I describe my system is changing and is in the process of changing. Sometimes I wonder if it's John the shell that is nothing without the other parts." Up until last fall there were four to five parts running the day-to-day show, although in his mind he had five to six other parts connected to those parts. He continues, "Every emotion takes a different personality to manage."

Contributors with a Previously Identified System Reporting Integration

As Amy Wagner said in her interview, "In our world, integration is an ugly word." While this is the case for most people I've met in the DID and dissociative disorders community, we have to be mindful not to project our triggers around the word onto others. Yes, integration in the classic sense can be described as bringing all of the parts together as a unified alloy. Even as I type this I wince, noting that I would never want that. Yet over the years of my own healing, our system has become more and more cooperative. This cooperation allows my brain to feel more integrated if we are defining integration as the brains of the triune brain working together. Remember, Dorothy needed all of her friends in *The Wizard of Oz* to help her to get home.

So it could be in our circles of healing that we may need to *redefine integration,* or, as we will do in this section, listen to the voices of contributors who describe themselves as having reached a sense of integration. For Dr. Kirsten Koenig, a Blackfeet therapist treated for an extensive complex and intergenerational trauma history, the language of system used to resonate for her, and she even had a metaphor. She explains, "I feel that I used to operate as a system for most of my adult life. I even likened my different faces to facets of a diamond. This always made me feel like the parts weren't a bad thing." Yet more recently, after a major life-threatening trauma described in chapter 3, she was able to accept the *parts of her* as *all of her.* Using another metaphor, she said that this was like knowing all the branches of her tree. She continued, "I went back and picked up my pieces, I had to find them, which means I had to feel them."

Dianne Harper, a spiritual director, aged sixty-four at the time of her interview, was diagnosed with DID thirty years ago. During her interview, she commented, "It's so cool to say that out loud to someone who knows what I'm talking about!" She said that in her healing, integrating the parts was not her original goal, although it gradually started to happen and to her knowledge, at this moment, she is fully integrated. In reflecting back, she remembers having six parts: another version of her pre-integration, the Center (a dancing and playful part who dissociated like "normal people do"), the Warrior (like the goddess Diana), the Good Girl (who came out whenever she needed to be compliant), the Wild Child (acting out), and Rose (her youngest part, who was the last to integrate).

Dianne explains, "Rose was very feral-like, she referred to herself as the secret keeper. Over time she became more beautiful and then one day, when I was about forty-seven, she was gone." When I asked her to elaborate, Dianne offered, "There was a hole in my brain and something was missing—that voice we were used to communicating with. It's not like I felt abandoned, though. I recognized she's part of who I am now."

In recalling her journey, Dianne reflects that once she got good at loving and honoring her parts, that's when they started to go away. And this transition came with much grief and loss for her that she also embraced. There are some, perhaps even some contributors to this book, who might read Dianne's story and still see her as a system. And it's very interesting that Dianne has full memory of them as a system yet is able to acknowledge the sense of integration that serves her and her life path. For Dianne it is not an either/or: "I don't really feel a need to say I'm integrated, no longer DID, or a working system. I just am who I am." My hope is that other readers of this book will be able to honor that for Dianne as well.

Empowering the Healing Path and Language We Choose

In this section, we conclude by discussing some of the controversies around terminology and our right to select the healing path and language that we choose. Many of our contributors, who fall into each category in the previous section, report that they are still learning about their systems and are not able to precisely articulate how they are formed. For six of our contributors, even though they identify as having parts or aspects of self, working to name them has not felt particularly necessary or helpful. In getting to know yourself and your relationship to dissociation, there is no pressure to fit into a certain mold. Even though people in this chapter have intricate knowledge of their systems or formations, please know that if this doesn't feel authentic for you, it is not required for engaging in healing work around dissociation and trauma. We hope that the variation here in how people with parts or systems describe them demonstrates how everything that feels authentic for you is on the table—even if that means seeing yourself as integrated or more integrated (although you may hear many people with DID discourage use of the word).

Amy Wagner has a sign in her clinical office that reads: "All Parts Welcome Here. No Parts Left Behind." Indeed, if you find yourself working with a therapist who tells you to ignore your parts or that you have to integrate in order to lead a deep and meaningful life, you are likely not in the best of hands. We honor that parts systems can take on various formations to help protect you and meet your needs. These parts may be fluid and change over time and with healing, and it's important that if you are seeking professional care that you seek out someone who is as nonpathologizing as possible and is willing to learn in collaboration with you.

There are a few comments about the wide world of parts in dissociation-informed care that are important to mention in conclusion. Several of our contributors did touch on pronouns, although in a very general way. As I mentioned in the introductory chapter, people with dissociative disorders and dissociative experiences of life may elect to use singular *we* and singular *they* pronouns to describe themselves. You're already aware that my system presents ourselves as *I* and *we* interchangeably. Issues around pronouns related to gender identity have received greater attention over the last decade and we in the dissociation community are happy about this movement away from making assumptions about how people identify and present themselves in the world. Moreover, many young people navigating their journey around gender identity might be experiencing parts of various genders. While we caution you that some more conservative people like to lean into the parts and dissociation explanation of gender expansion instead of accepting that a loved one might be sorting out issues around gender identity and expression, an interplay can exist. So if you are a reader navigating issues around your dissociation, parts, and gender identity, seeking someone qualified to help you sort it all out is advisable. Or if that is not an option right now, please continue being kind to yourself and know that you are in charge of how you identify.

Sandra Johnson, one of our contributors with DID, offered one sentence in her interview that said so much: "In my own words there is so much expansion behind the *I*, but I use it to hide so much." Perhaps you are a plural system and you've thought about using *we/they* pronouns but have been afraid to try them out in any public way. You can begin by writing in that way, even if it's in a journal for yourself and notice how that feels for you; or start trying it out with your therapist or any close friends who know about your plurality. Using *we* or *they* pronouns is also not a requirement to address dissociation in a clinical sense or even in a general sense. We just want to mention it here as a further validation of what some of you may be experiencing.

Another note is that many systems identify as containing multiple genders (some of them are described by our contributors like Megan), species (recall Elizabeth Davis's dog part, and Alexis's parts each having animal or mythical creatures protecting them), or races and ethnic backgrounds. Often, connection with a member of another racial or ethnic background could be related to past life belief systems; or strong relationships with characters of that racial or ethnic background in folklore, movies/television, fiction, or even in real life. System formations across genders, species, and races/ethnicities are all plausible. However, the consultation I've received from persons of color within the dissociation community is that if you are a white person or member of the dominant culture who has a part or parts who are non-white or part of an oppressed group that you are not born into, it is important that you do not claim to be an expert on the lived experience of that group in the world. Recognize that as a white person, or perhaps as a straight person who identifies as having a queer part, you still maintain a great deal of privilege, and suggesting otherwise is insulting to a marginalized group. If you want to take your engagement with your parts a step further, it may be vitally important for your healing to learn about the oppressions experienced by a part you identify who is not of your race, sexual orientation, or other identifier.

The two main reasons I've seen many white people develop non-white parts and straight people develop queer parts is the connection with being treated poorly in the world. Sometimes there is a strong sense of experiencing a past life as a person from another place or experience of life. And yes, while I realize the mere mention of *past lives* may further bring some of you out of your comfort zones, please be aware that many of our contributors and folks with dissociative experiences of life do feel connection to their parts through past lives. If this is not a part of your personal belief system or theology, once more, you do not have to adopt it. However, be mindful that the belief systems of most of the world allow for some teaching on the cycle of death and rebirth. As Julian Jaramillo, one of our Shamanic contributors, may caution, "Be mindful of your privileged way of looking at reality."

There are many, many more parts formations that can exist beyond what our contributors offered here. In the Recommended Reading and Resources section we provide a wide collection of memoirs and creative fiction, based on contributors' dissociative experiences, that you can investigate further. The only caution I would give you in reading some of these is that many of the descriptions of traumatic experiences in the memoirs can be graphic, as opposed to most of the vignettes and stories shared in this book that do not focus as much on the trauma itself. You are the empowered navigator of your own recovery, so you might find reading some of these memoirs a logical next step after the skill foundations you've established in working through this book.

EXPRESSIVE ARTS PRACTICE: THE PARTS MAPPING EXERCISE

Remember that you do not have to qualify for a dissociative disorder or any mental health issue to identify, name, and map your parts. Even the words you choose, as evidenced by some of the contributor insights in this chapter, are variable. Instead of *parts* you may elect to use the words *selves, roles, aspects, people,* or any other concept that seems to fit. Instead of a *system* perhaps a word like *constellation, collective,* or *dimensions* works for you.

How would you "map" your internal world? If the idea of a literal map works for you, either like a map of states and countries or a road map, go with it! Perhaps some of the other metaphors in this chapter struck a chord; or you may have been inspired by what you read in this chapter and thought of a metaphor, a mythology, a literary world, or a cinematic universe that works better for you. In addition to some of the metaphors listed in this chapter, you are also welcome to borrow some others that people I've worked with and taught have also implemented: a bouquet of flowers, a bunch of balloons, a stew with various ingredients (salads also work), instruments in a band or an orchestra, keys on a key ring, mosaics, rooms of a house, the car or van (my personal favorite), or sitting in a circle as in group therapy or a meeting.

This project might evolve over the course of several days or weeks and it is not meant to be diagnostic in nature. This exercise is intended to be an exploration that can inform your current therapy or healing, or it may inspire you to seek out a more formal consultation with a therapist or other qualified healing professional. As always, take great care to step away and attend to your grounding needs if any part of this exercise becomes too overwhelming. You have complete permission to be as simple or intricately detailed as you would like with this exercise. Perhaps you keep it on a page or in your journal, or you may elect to get three-dimensional and crafty with it. Crystal, one of our contributors, avidly makes glass mosaics that show a very detailed respect for parts and system. So while you do not have to spend a lot of money on this project, if your visual artist is wanting to come out, let them come out to play! As an alternative, you can visit the playlist exercise from the previous chapter again and consider mapping your system as a playlist.

⸺QUESTIONS TO ASK MY THERAPIST OR PSYCHIATRIST⸺

- What is your general approach to working with parts? Do you use one model, a series of models, or no particular model?
- Do you believe that all people have an internal system of some kind? If so, tell me more about how you see systems.

- What are your feelings about integration of parts? Are you open to using other words or concepts besides *integration?*

- How do you handle the voices and experiences of parts that seem to be most responsible for causing problems or acting out in my life?

- What has been your experience so far in working with parts or a system in someone who is like me? Are you willing to get consultation if you feel stuck?

- What are your feelings about integrating my spiritual beliefs, or beliefs not easily explained by the laws of science, into our healing process?

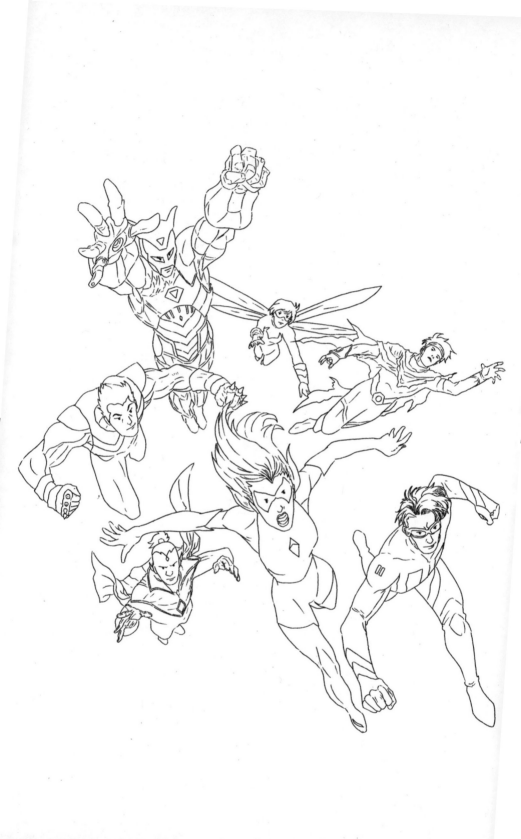

5

The Dissociative Profile

Just as a prism reflects light differently when you change its angle, each experience of love illuminates love in new ways, drawing from an infinite pattern of palettes and hues.

—SHARON SALZBERG

Many teachers describe dissociation as a continuum phenomenon. We all dissociate, some more than others, and the experience may manifest differently at different times depending upon the nature and intensity of stressors. On the "mild" end of the continuum, the behaviors that every human being can experience, like daydreaming or losing attention while driving, are presented. DID and other dissociative disorders can appear on the "extreme" end of the continuum. A person or system may fluctuate on the continuum depending on where they are *at* during any given time in their life in response to trauma, loss, and stress.

As I first contended in my major coming-out article from 2018,[1] the continuum can be a good start when you're first learning about dissociation. Yet for me/us the continuum construct is too linear. I regard dissociation as prismatic. Light flows through a prism to reflect a series of colors—the more angles on a prism, the more dramatically light splits as it comes through—resulting in fascinatingly complex and stunningly beautiful patterns and fractals. For a prism to be a prism, at least two angles made of material transparent to the wavelengths of light for which they are designed must exist. Some folks have two angles, others have hundreds. The more intense the light (which can be a metaphor for life stressors), the more radiant the reflection. For those of us who have learned how the angles of our prism serve us under stress, *radiant* is an ideal adjective. Prior to our learning how they work, the dispersion of light can feel blinding and confusing, to us and to others in our lives. Shutting down the prism altogether can seem more appealing. When we go offline, or any connection to affect or emotion goes out the window, it can be a sign of such a shutdown or desire to withdraw.

We've already established in this book that dissociation can be many things in many contexts. You may find that, after noticing what you've discovered about yourself so far, that the continuum description may resonate for you. Something like the prism, or another metaphorical description altogether may work best. The objective of this chapter is to take what you've discovered in this book so far and construct what I call your Dissociative Profile. The Dissociative Profile is a dynamic exercise that challenges us to evaluate and be aware of one's own tendencies to dissociate, both adaptively and maladaptively. In this investigation, we also identify the best strategies for directing one's knowing awareness back to here-and-now presence. This exercise is not only valuable as an exploratory device. The knowledge you take from it will become a valuable part of developing your own plan for healing, which may or may not involve psychotherapy. In the event you are involved with therapy or another professional healing modality, knowing the intricacies of your dissociative profile can help you manage distress that may rise in between sessions.

Your Dissociative Profile may change over time. My system and I engage in the exercise in this chapter at least once a year, or during major life changes. The Dissociative Profile is an endeavor in self-study. Now is the most appropriate time in the book for us to introduce this practice, since you've received a great deal of foundational material up to this point, and you have hopefully completed or are working on some type of parts mapping. Having an awareness of your system can allow you to more fully engage in this exercise, although as established in the prior chapter, having a precisely defined system is not a requirement for doing this work.

Before taking you through the instructions for investigating your Dissociative Profile and putting it down on paper, there are two concepts that we will unpack. In trauma-informed and trauma-focused studies, the Window of Tolerance model, as introduced by Dr. Daniel Siegel, is a widely accepted model for tracking intensity and one's ability to be present with it. However, for many of us with dissociative disorders, the Window of Tolerance model is not only too linear, it is not sufficiently dimensional. Although many people will find the Window of Tolerance model useful in constructing their Dissociative Profiles, you may prefer instead to use a more dimensional model created by Katarina Lundgren, one of our contributors, called the Wheel of Tolerance. In this chapter, we devote an entire section to exploring the differences between the two models. Then, before formally guiding you on how to put together your Dissociative Profile, we will further explore the construct of intersectionality and how it may apply to your identity/identities as you engage in your self-study. Finally we will move into best practices for putting together your Dissociative Profile, offer you some examples of what they can look like, and further discuss how it can inform the healing path ahead.

The Window of Tolerance versus the Wheel of Tolerance

As the name of the Window of Tolerance model[2] suggests, when a person is in their *window,* they are able to stay present with sensation and affect or emotion in a way that is not harmful to them. Widely accepted among trauma educators, the Window of Tolerance model can be a useful tool in helping a person determine if they are in a safe enough zone to handle working with deeper, more emotionally charged material. When it's working at its best, the person and their treating clinician can use the window of tolerance language to determine best courses of action in treatment, and for developing skills to expand the metaphorical window. Some people have larger windows of tolerance than others, and through therapy and other healing practices, people can learn to expand their window of tolerance. When a window of tolerance is wide, an individual or their system is able to handle the navigation of stressors, triggers, and emotional distress that may emerge in therapy without going into a potentially dangerous hyperarousal (too much) or hypoarousal (too little/withdrawn) state. The model contends that a healthy nervous system maintains an appropriate degree of sympathetic (arousal) and parasympathetic (rest and digest) balance to allow an individual to manage the emotional triggers of life. When one is in their window of tolerance, they tend to interact more effectively in relationships, have a greater capacity to be psychologically flexible, and more gracefully meet daily challenges. Bringing in the polyvagal theory covered in chapter 2, we are generally in a ventral vagal state when we are in our affective window of tolerance.

Window of Tolerance

Hyperarousal

Sympathetic nervous system:

Mobilization with fear

Fight or Flight

Survival & Protection Mode

Dysregulation

Unsafe

Too much energy
Increase in heart rate

Reactive/ Chaos
- Anger
- Defensive
- Explosive
- Screaming
- Anxious
- No care for consequences
- Rage
- Disregard or aggression towards others

Mobilization with safety (without fear)

Engage in behaviors that demand activity, friendly competition, excitement, exercise

Window Of Tolerance

Parasympathetic nervous system:

Ventral vagal social engagement / Communication

Optimal arousal zone

Thriving & Connection mode

Regulation

Safe

Optimal energy

Clarity in thinking and focus

Resilience

Receptive
- Love
- Joy
- Compassion
- Patience
- Aware of self, others and surrounding
- Curious
- Problem solving
- Considers consequences

Mobilization with safety (without fear)

Engage in behaviors that don't demand excess activity: nuturing, quiet social connection

Hypoarousal

Parasympathetic nervous system:

Dorsal Vagal Immobilization with fear

Freeze

Survival & Protection mode

Dysregulation

Unsafe

Too little or lack of energy
Decrease in heart rate

Reactive/ Rigidity
- Slow
- Exhausted
- Slow
- Giving up
- Shut down
- Numb
- Dissociation
- Resignation
- Low muscle tone
- Disconnect from others
- Apathy
- Collapse

The more a person or system's brain is trying to manage, the more likely we are to be thrown off balance, or knocked out of our ideal middle window. An excess of sympathetic activation can cause a person to go past or over their affective window of tolerance. This state is called hyperarousal, commonly associated with the flight/fight response. Common signs of hyperarousal include being anxious, easily overwhelmed, easily angered, prone to outbursts or aggression. Other signs of hyperarousal may include any variety of acting out behaviors (e.g., excessive drinking, drug use, overeating), mental rigidity, or obsessive–compulsive thoughts and behaviors. This state and these behaviors also align with how polyvagal theory describes the sympathetic nervous system.

Another possibility is that the balance can be tipped the other way toward hypoarousal, or an excess of parasympathetic activation. While some freeze responses (think "deer in the headlights") might have a quality of hyperarousal (a freeze that also comes with some activation like heart racing), a response called freeze to submission and the immobility that comes with it can be framed as a hypoarousal. Other responses of hypoarousal can include fawning, collapsing, or otherwise shutting down. Examples may include depressive tendencies or flat affect, memory loss, feeling disconnected, operating on autopilot, and feeling separated from the self or otherwise not present. In the language of polyvagal theory, this experience is dorsal vagal in nature.

Some teachers in somatic psychology will use the metaphor of a light switch to explain the Window of Tolerance model. Hyperarousal responses are like having a light switch constantly "on," and hypoarousal is being stuck with the switch "off." A healthy system needs a balance of the two, and unhealed trauma can make living in this balance difficult. Therapists who work in a variety of modalities and systems make use of the Window of Tolerance model. We teach people to recognize that when they are in hyperarousal they will need to down-regulate to come back into the ideal window. Engaging in more action-based behaviors like light exercise, playfulness, or even games can be ideal for this process of literally shaking off or loosening the excess activation. When a person is in a hypoaroused response, grounding, quiet, and activities that create a sense of nurturing and connection are ideal to return to the window of tolerance and thus a ventral vagal response.

This model may make perfect sense to you, and as you complete your Dissociative Profile it may be useful to frame your questions as, "What will bring me back into my affective window of tolerance if I am dissociated, otherwise hypoaroused, or even hyperaroused?" Yet for many of us with complex trauma, dissociative disorders, and dissociative experiences of life, the Window of Tolerance model can feel too linear and too simplistic. Many of us with dissociative tendencies, experiences, and diagnoses report being able to experience states of hyperarousal and hypoarousal at the same time—at least it can seem that way if two or more parts or aspects of our experience are activated simultaneously. I also can experience being in a hyperaroused state and then immediately drop into a hypoaroused state characterized by serious dissociative collapse without ever passing through that middle window. I can also experience and present being fully in my ventral vagal state, connected and engaged with my therapist or others around me . . . and I can be crying excessively or feel like I'm otherwise jumping out of my skin. An outside observer or a therapist who doesn't know my system and me well might assume this means I'm outside my window and not okay to work on stuff. Yet knowing myself (and thankfully my therapist, Elizabeth, knows me well), these states are often when I am in the best position to therapeutically engage with my emotions and sensations.

Katarina Lundgren, the Swedish equine therapist with DID, is not impressed by many of the models in the psychotherapeutic arena, even in those circles that claim to be more trauma-focused. So many of the models that are out there, she says, "feel like complete B.S. and are clueless about dissociation." Katarina, in turn, made a proposal of her own on her blog about a more dimensional way to look at activation and collapse. Instead of a linear continuum or a vertically-oriented window model, she turned to the shape of a circle.

When Katarina explained to me her idea of the Wheel of Tolerance in our interview, my entire system pinged with a sense of deep resonance.

"This makes so much more sense to us," I told her, "especially as someone who feels that I can be in fight and freeze at the same time!"

Katarina explains, "When you're in the center of your wheel of tolerance, you're pretty composed. And then when something happens, you may move out, and it becomes like a spiderweb. You may spread out in the direction of fight, flight, freeze, or fawn, at least as I see it. When you're spread out in a lot of directions, you are prone to dissociate."

You can see the attached images, shared with Katarina's permission, on how someone's wheel of tolerance might present if they are being pulled in several directions. As Katarina explains on her diagram, the closer one might be to the center, the more likely they are to be in their fullest experience of Self. This state comes close to what is traditionally seen as being in the affective window of tolerance.

Wheel of Tolerance

FIGHT
Hit, scream, brace, abuse, lash out,
be sarcastic, dark humor, bully,
dominate . . .

FLIGHT
Run, hide, "spin," fidget/stim,
daydream, imagine, books/films,
rationalize, dissociate . . .

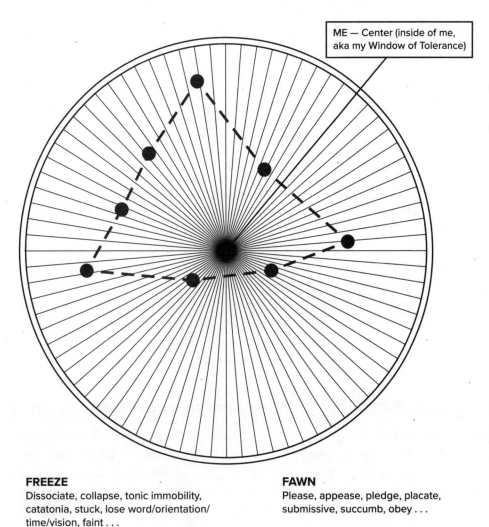

ME — Center (inside of me,
aka my Window of Tolerance)

FREEZE
Dissociate, collapse, tonic immobility,
catatonia, stuck, lose word/orientation/
time/vision, faint . . .

FAWN
Please, appease, pledge, placate,
submissive, succumb, obey . . .

In the original 2019 article Katarina wrote on the Wheel of Tolerance model, she calls for us having a more nuanced discussion than the current trauma models are allowing us to have. Katarina expresses in this piece a common frustration that many people with dissociative minds experience when we go to therapy with someone who doesn't seem to grasp how multidimensional we can be. She asks:

> Isn't it possible for all people to be in several emotional states at once? Have several emotions or feelings at once? Like being scared, but feeling joyful at the same time? Feeling curious, but upset at the same time? Feeling scared, joyful, curious and upset at the same time? Even having more contradictory emotions at the same time—feeling love and hate at the same time? Fear and relaxation? Anger and content? What is the difference then if you are in a stress or trauma response? Aren't they emotional states as well? Is it only highly dissociative people who can be in flight and freeze at the same time? Or move between them—several times—in a traumatic situation—as well as in working with traumatic material?[3]

Having multiple feelings and states of experience at once, especially in response to trauma and stress, we feel, is normal. As people with dissociative minds, Katarina and I know this to be possible, and it's something we wish to affirm for others as well as a perfectly reasonable response to trauma and stress.

So in preparing to begin and complete your *Dissociative Profile* Exercise, you may consider contemplating the Window of Tolerance model versus the Wheel of Tolerance model to see which one resonates best for you and, if applicable, your system. When the *Dissociative Profile* Exercise asks you to contemplate which skills or strategies might be best for returning you to the present moment or the here and now, you can also conceptualize that invitation as "Which skills or strategies help to bring you into your window of tolerance or closer to the center of your wheel of tolerance?"

Intersectionality and Connections to Dissociation

Intersectionality is a term coined by Black feminist legal scholar Kimberlé Williams Crenshaw in 1989. Primarily used in law and social justice discourse, intersectionality and intersectional analysis consider a collection of factors that affect the individual in combination, rather than considering the factors in isolation.[4] What started as an obscure legal term has now entered more of our mainstream discourse, with many conservative critics claiming that it's just a way for people to capitalize on all of the manners in which they've been victimized by the mainstream. You can read many excellent articles and interviews from Crenshaw herself on intersectionality via a simple Internet search, where she discusses what intersectionality is and isn't. One of my

favorite explanations she gives connects beautifully to my thoughts on dissociation as explored at the beginning of this chapter:

> Intersectionality was a prism to bring to light dynamics within discrimination
> law that weren't being appreciated by the courts. In particular, courts seem to
> think that race discrimination was what happened to all black people across
> gender and sex discrimination was what happened to all women, and if that is
> your framework, of course, what happens to black women and other women
> of color is going to be difficult to see.[5]

Once more, the prism shines light where society has traditionally attempted
to see things only through simplified labels.

To evaluate where intersectionality may apply to you as you prepare to
develop your *Dissociative Profile* Exercise, consider going back to the Intersections Venn diagram practice from chapter 2. Did you bring in any aspects of
your identity in that exercise that may feel relevant to this discussion? In what
ways might some of your identities, such as being a person of color, being a
woman, being disabled, or your sexual orientation or gender identity—and
the discrimination you may experience based on any of these identities—feel
like they might complicate the healing process for you? Might the compounding factors, any of which can be evidence of the dissociation that mainstream
society can promote to keep power structures in play, create more of a need
in you to cope with dissociation? Sometimes this might happen consciously,
sometimes it can feel like you've been dissociating for so long just to stay
afloat, you might not even recognize that you're doing it. If any of these barriers exist for you or feel especially difficult for your parts to navigate, consider
how they might show up in the *Dissociative Profile* Exercise to follow.

THE DISSOCIATIVE PROFILE EXERCISE

Before engaging in this exercise, please remember that every human being
dissociates. This is *not* an exercise in shaming, rather an invitation into self-
inquiry. Here are the general steps we recommend for beginning to investigate
and compose your Dissociative Profile. This first set of instructions assumes
a basic Dissociative Profile for an individual without a significantly defined
parts system, and a sample Dissociative Profile follows. Then, we will go into
offering ideas for creating a more intricate Dissociative Profile assuming the
existence of a more defined system with multiple parts.

BASIC DISSOCIATIVE PROFILE

- Take out some paper or open up a word processing program on your computer.

- Make two columns. Title the left-hand column "My Dissociative Tendencies," and title the right-hand column, "What Helps Me Return to the Present Moment."

- Take as much time as you need to make a list of the ways in which you tend to dissociate or separate from present-moment awareness. You can note general patterns like "zoning out or daydreaming when I'm bored," or "spending too much time on Facebook or TikTok and wondering what everyone else is doing."

- You can take this inventory a step further by noting if these strategies or behaviors are adaptive, maladaptive, or both (depending on context). Also note, perhaps, how often you engage in these dissociative strategies and whether you have knowing awareness about what sets them off or triggers them (e.g., boredom, emotional pain, overwhelm, conversations with certain people).

- After the left-hand side feels complete, go to the right-hand column and beside each item on the left, make some notes about what helps you return to the present moment when you need to. Remember, another way to think of this return can be to the window of tolerance or to the center of the wheel of tolerance. These skills can be more intrinsic (e.g., grounding by holding a solid object in my hand, taking a mindful walk), or more externally motivating factors (e.g., hearing my child call out that they need me, hearing the phone ring). Be honest and note if you are not yet sure how to draw yourself back to present moment awareness when you get stuck in certain patterns.

- After finishing your own Dissociative Profile, notice whatever you notice. Is there anything in your columns that surprises you? Is there anything you might consider sharing with your own therapist, a friend, a partner, or members of your support system? How can you use what you discover here to assist you in your own personal development and goals or intentions for healing? Consider taking some time to freewrite or journal on these questions, quietly contemplate them, or use them as a basis of conversation with your therapist, healing professional, or a trusted friend.

SAMPLE DISSOCIATIVE PROFILE EXERCISE (BASIC)

MY DISSOCIATIVE TENDENCIES	WHAT HELPS ME RETURN TO THE PRESENT MOMENT
Daydreaming when I'm bored—this was helpful (adaptive) when I was a kid, it's how I survived my parents' constant fighting. Somewhat of a problem/maladaptive now as it can keep me from paying attention at work.	Telling myself to "snap out of it" helps sometimes; this is something I'd like to work on, though, because it can be hard to get out of the dream world. Recently discovered that smelling some peppermint oil or sucking on a peppermint candy can also be helpful to bring me out of the daydream. Doodling or drawing what can feel like nonsense on a page is also helpful.
Watching too many TikTok videos on the phone—boredom also seems to trigger this. Doesn't seem to be a problem at the level of addiction or anything; I just know I do it too much, when it's probably healthier for me to do something like take a walk.	Sometimes my eyes get too strained or tired and that helps me put the phone down; or when I know I have something more exciting/stimulating to work on. This can include having a conversation with people I enjoy.
Saying "it's no big deal" to my own therapist whenever I get too emotional or teary; it's clear that this protected me at home growing up (adaptive) yet I know it gets in the way of me working on what I know I could be working on in therapy. It's almost become a joke between my therapist and me now that saying "it's no big deal" is a sign that something really is "a big deal."	Having my therapist, whom I usually trust, gently call me out on my tendency to do this seems to help. Sometimes she just has to give me a look that is caring yet shows she is also challenging me. When she can guide me through one of her mindfulness exercises and encourage me to notice my body and be with whatever is coming up, I make steps in the right direction. Sometimes it's easier to stand up in these moments instead of sit down.
Problems paying attention when I drive (only sometimes)—I'm not sure if this is dissociation or just general distraction. Either way, it does seem to happen when I'm overwhelmed or have had a stressful day at work.	Playing music I like in the car helps. I haven't yet tried my therapist's suggestion of taking a few deep breaths before I start driving, regardless of how I'm feeling. Seems like a good idea to try that.

═SYSTEM OR MULTIDIMENSIONAL DISSOCIATIVE PROFILE═

People with an awareness of their parts or with refined systems might be all over the place, metaphorically speaking, in the presence of a stressor or trigger because different parts have different experiences of that stressor or trigger. Hence, we are fans of Katarina Lundgren's Wheel of Tolerance model because it allows for mapping experience in a more multidimensional way. Something that upsets one part might feel like no big deal to the others.

One of the reasons I placed the parts chapter with the *Parts Mapping* Exercise before the *Dissociative Profile* Exercise is so you can play with the same fundamental Dissociative Profile introduced in the section above. Now make some more notes as they may relate to your parts, your selves, and your inner world. We encourage you to keep as open and curious of a mind and heart space as possible as you engage in this version of the Dissociative Profile with your parts. In naming a trigger for dissociation and unpacking its meaning, you might discover that one of your parts has a solution for you that you'd never previously considered.

As with the *Parts Mapping* Exercise in the previous chapter, there is no pressure to do this exercise all in one sitting. You can let things unfold over the course of a week or so and perhaps engage in some inventory at the end of each evening to notice what you notice. Myself and others have also been known to use a strategy like, "Team, what do you need me/us to know about working with this trigger or this issue that we haven't previously seen before?" Some free writing to address this question might be in order before you begin this version of the *Dissociative Profile* Exercise.

SAMPLE DISSOCIATIVE PROFILE EXERCISE (SYSTEM)

MY/OUR DISSOCIATIVE TENDENCIES	WHAT HELPS ME/US RETURN TO THE PRESENT MOMENT
Closing our eyes or looking away whenever our partner looks at us romantically for too long (even though most of us like this, it can scare our youngest part and make our teenage part think that because our partner loves us, things will inevitably go wrong).	External: Having our partner ask us, "Where did you just go?" or "Is there anything I'm missing here?" Internal: Drawing our attention to or touching the third eye, the place in the center of our forehead. Or allowing our adult part to whisper to our youngest part and our teenage part that our partner is a safe person for us.

MY/OUR DISSOCIATIVE TENDENCIES	WHAT HELPS ME/US RETURN TO THE PRESENT MOMENT
Having our boss at work raise her voice at us; our youngest part feels like she's being punished and the teenage part wants to go into fighting mode. So we just click into this autopilot mode and smile and nod; feels adaptive as it keeps us from getting fired but we can feel gross afterward.	Taking a breath and drawing our attention to the third eye (center of the forehead) seems to help all of us at the same time. Can help us ride out the experience and dissociate only minimally. After our boss leaves, it's helpful for us to visualize going to our internal conference table and having a meeting so that we can all be heard. This strategy works on that same day although we know we also need to report it to our therapist the next time we see them. Listening to music in our office if possible at some point that day will help, at least on the drive home from work.
Seeing something upsetting on the news that involves people being mistreated by the system or government; can make us zone out but in a way where we still feel our blood boil as we get very angry, especially as a queer woman who has been mistreated by the mental health system.	On some days we need to turn off the news and go outside and take a walk or at least go outside and get some air if our body is starting to feel too uncomfortable. Our teenage/angry part and protector are often helped by drinking some cold water or having an ice pack on their head while they watch the news. Our idealist part likes to do a yoga stretch or say a prayer—she can do this while she watches the news and feel okay since staying informed is important to her.
Listening to our own children (our external children, not our children inside) fight with each other; when it gets too overwhelming, can sound like they are talking in nonsense like Charlie Brown's mom, or like they are at the other side of a tunnel. Allowing their voices to fog out like that feels	During the moment of their fighting, pressing our feet into the ground seems to help all of our parts. Calling for the dog to be near me/ us during these fights, if possible, is helpful—making contact with her fur keeps us there.

(continues)

SAMPLE DISSOCIATIVE PROFILE EXERCISE (SYSTEM) *(continued)*

MY/OUR DISSOCIATIVE TENDENCIES	WHAT HELPS ME/US RETURN TO THE PRESENT MOMENT
adaptive or helpful most times, or I might go off on them!	After their fighting we also need to meet at our internal conference table and listen to what our youngest parts have to say about how our external children upset them. If possible, the other parts and I will all need to do something fun for the younger part later that night. Having an ice cream cone can help if watching a movie that the younger part likes isn't helpful.

If completing this version of the Dissociative Profile feels like a better fit for you, or if your first Dissociative Profile organically turned out this way, consider reflecting on the following questions:

- Is there anything in your columns that surprises you?
- Is there anything you might consider sharing with your own therapist, a friend, a partner, or members of your support system?
- How can you use what you discover here to assist you in your own personal development and goals or intentions for healing?

Consider taking some time to freewrite or journal on these questions, quietly contemplate them, or use them as a basis of conversation with your therapist, healing professional, or a trusted friend. As always, the different parts of your system may chime in with their opinions and perspectives. If that happens and the system feels safe enough to continue exploring, keep going with whatever comes up in your writing or other expression.

PARTS SCENE WORK EXPLORATION

This next exercise asks you to take the parts mapping you did in the previous chapter and engage with it a little further. Now that you have a basic map and have done a version of the Dissociative Profile, this exercise will hopefully have more meaning and really come to life for you and your system. After completing this exercise—which, like all of our exercises, you can allow to evolve over time—you may consider returning to your Dissociative Profile and making relevant tweaks based on new insights gained here.

The purpose of this exercise is to further explore how your internal world or system communicates with each other. By engaging in this exploration, we can identify what areas of further inquiry and communication may need to take place.

- Take a look at what you created in your *Parts Mapping* Exercise. Is there one part, segment, or facet of it that grabs your attention the most? If so, notice it and consider the question: If that part had a message for me right now, what would it be? It is totally permissible to use the presenting adult/core ego state/ANP/Self if that is what you are noticing the most. Take about three to five minutes to freewrite.

- After this initial writing, look at the parts map once more and notice if there is a second part that is also calling for your attention. Same thing—notice it and ask, if that part had a message for me right now, what would it be? Take about three to five minutes to freewrite.

- Now write a dialogue between the two parts or aspects of self. Take at least three to five minutes to let this dialogue unfold, although you may take longer if you wish. Consider using the following style, as if you were writing a scene in a play:

ADULT JAMIE (AJ) *I'm working on my presentation for the EMDR conference.*

9 *Oh boy, you still go to that?*

AJ *Of course. It's gotten better for me. For all of us, I think.*

9 *What are you teaching on this year?*

AJ *Dissociation—about how our mind works.*

9 *Oh brother. Do you think we can handle it without chewing their heads off?*

AJ *I'm hoping we can. Can I get your input first?*

9 *You really sure you want to hear from me on this one?*

AJ *Yes I do.*

- You can name your parts or aspects of self whatever you wish. If working with age or names of specific parts doesn't seem to be a good fit, you can use emotions or other places in your life where you seem to notice separation. As another example, here is a small scene that flowed out in some of my writing as I invited my human self and my Divine Self into dialogue with each other:

HUMAN *This sucks!*

DIVINE *I know.*

HUMAN *Do you? Do you really?*

DIVINE *Go on . . . I want to hear about it.*

- As with every exercise we've done thus far in this course, do not censor yourself. Go with whatever unfolds, being open to any surprises or insights. If at any point you feel too overwhelmed, you have complete permission to pause and go back to one of your grounding or other coping skills. You can choose to resume the exercise later or leave it be. Consider going over any insights later with a therapist, another healing professional, or a trusted friend.

Parts scene work, which I sometimes call parts journaling, is a particular favorite skill of mine. In my own therapeutic work, it is a powerful exercise for helping my system take care of themselves in between therapy sessions, and many of my clients find this exercise useful for this reason. Although I advise writing between two parts or aspects to begin, of course the voices of other parts can be brought in to the scene. These other parts or aspects may create a mediating influence or hold an important part of the solution for the system around areas of conflict or disagreement.

As is the way of things in expressive arts therapy, engaging in one form like writing can open up invitations to introduce other expressive forms, to further bring the exercise to life. For some people, after they engage in the parts journaling, it can feel nourishing and transformative to make art (even if it's scribbles or doodles) on top of the words. With any kind of journaling, you do not need to leave your words hanging around and exposed for others to see. While ripping up or safely burning what you write are always options, you may find it even more transformative to make new art on top of writing that no longer serves you. If working with movement, consider this practice: If one part's message could be expressed in a movement or a gesture, what would that be? Then notice: If the other part's message could be expressed in a movement or a gesture, what would that gesture be? Spend a few minutes going back and forth between the movements/gestures and see what naturally unfolds in your movement or dance.

Making the Dissociative Profile and Self-Study Work for You

The *Dissociative Profile* Exercises in this chapter are meant to give you some ideas, not be absolute models or systems that you have to follow. We hope you've received some ideas for noticing whether the continuum or the prism examples that opened the chapter work best for you to understand yourself. Maybe you've thought of some combination of the two that works better, or something altogether different? Does the idea of a Window of Tolerance or Wheel of Tolerance model seem like a better fit in helping you track how you respond to life, and learn what you might need to return to some form of center or balance so you can most healthfully engage with life? And perhaps the two columns of the Dissociative Profile that I offered feel too limiting. Is there another way you can track or map some of your triggers and responses, and what it might take to come back to center? Be sure to visit the expressive arts practice at the end of the chapter for some more ideas.

Whether you use any of the formal exercises presented in this chapter or develop some of your own, learning to listen to signals and coming to know yourself and your system will help you navigate a world full of triggers in the most adaptive way possible for you. Moreover, being able to work with your own patterns and skills like this on your own time can be imperative for getting the most out of therapy or any other professional healing art. A good trauma therapist will take caution to ensure that you have a reasonable set of skills and strategies you can use in between your therapy sessions, especially if a previous session was intense. We have a recognition that life, especially if you are living around a great deal of trauma and stress, can continue to cause dissociative responses or bring about upheaval in your system or your internal world in general. So if a therapist takes you into what feels like deeper work without having an in-between-session plan in place, be cautious or advocate for yourself about developing one.

Another reason we've placed this chapter before the following chapter on methods for deeper healing and connection is to emphasize that this preparation and awareness ideally come before taking the journey further into areas of more intense emotion and body sensation. Yet in this spirit of *nothing is linear,* recognize that if you end up engaging in deeper therapeutic or healing work and are feeling unsteady, consider coming back to your Dissociative Profile and examine it again. What might need to be changed or altered? Are there additional skills that you or some of your parts might need to build in order to feel better about exploring a certain area of your story? How might engaging with a greater sense of communication with your system reveal what might be missing? Remember that you can bring in any insights from the parts scene work in reexamining your Dissociative Profile.

To formally conclude this chapter, we turn to the words of our contributors and what they revealed about the process of *knowing thyself* in their healing. Two of our contributors, TaNiya and Cheryl, directly used the word *stubborn* to describe their systems. For them, that's a good thing. This stubbornness and tenacity facilitates their desire to learn about their system, its patterns, and its responses. And for Cheryl, embracing an attitude of trial and error helps her in learning about what is useful to her system and optimal for her process. For Danyale Weems, being a therapist herself and having a thirst for knowledge has helped her make connections about her own healing and the work she needs to do. Jackson feels similarly, noting that reading about his own trauma through study is a life raft, seeing this practice as even more essential as society and democracy unravel. John Fugett describes himself as someone who can be fundamentally dissociated and grounded at the same time. Yet being able to figure out what was really going on with his responses to life as indicative of a dissociative disorder was relieving. "It made sense in every way," said John.

Adam O'Brien recognizes that at times in his life, there has been safety in his chaos. Crystal also recognizes, with great awareness of herself and her patterns, "There are some times I don't want to be grounded. I just want to be safe and comfortable." Alexis notes, in sharing what she's learned about herself, "Even when I am going three steps back, I am progressing." Such an attitude has allowed her and her system to be less self-critical and fundamentally more embracing of their healing path.

For Rebecca, learning to ask simple questions like, "What feels helpful? And what feels harmful?" is critical in conducting self-inquiry. Malika has learned to ask a question like, "What is the empowered solution here?" And when she can identify it, she suddenly feels safe. Dr. Kirsten Koenig expresses, "I've learned that self-care is learning to love yourself as much as you were trained to love others." A.J. recalls that once—when being open to what parts will reveal—she was able to identify an emerging part as anger, feel it, and then the part was gone.

Jacqueline Lucas recognizes that when she needs to make big decisions in her life, checking in with all of her parts can be important. In our experience, engaging in parts scene work or journaling can be a powerful tool in doing such a check-in. The Garden System, who's developed a great understanding of how they operate, has a recognition that some of their parts show up for their professional work life and others don't. For Heather (LS) Scarboro+, who presents with a very finessed understanding of their system, a sense of compromise is needed for optimal functioning. Heather (LS+) describes compromise as a state where everyone feels heard and validated, and being in denial in any way can block this compromise. They further reflect, "For us, DID has been a practice to maintain awareness, even when we're fluid with who is present."

Self-inquiry (or system inquiry) can be an important part of the healing process and is imperative in dissociation recovery if you desire to engage with the world in the most adaptive way possible. Through their interviews our contributors suggest that there are many ways to engage this process and it's most important to identify what works. How do you know something is working? Generally, when there's a sense that you're feeling better or feeling more present and grounded in your ability to engage with life. Yet even defining how something is working in your life and within your system is subjective. As we'll explore in the next chapter, this process of growth and healing can take on many forms. Hopefully the strategies we covered in this chapter will allow you to have a foundation and several practice anchors for checking in with yourself and examining what is working as you move ahead in your healing.

EXPRESSIVE ARTS PRACTICE: WORKING WITH COLORS, SYMBOLS, AND CUES

If you recall in chapter 2, we explained that neuroception is allowing your body to recognize that something is wrong ten steps before your rational mind even realizes it. Learning to be cognizant at this body level is one of the many reasons I am sober today, and a main reason that my dissociative tendencies no longer reach the level of completely destroying me. Many people truly feel they have no choice but to dissociate in the presence of stress—that it's subconscious or automatic. And for most of us, dissociation is just that . . . at first. Yet once we have the recognition of what our patterns are, we may feel more empowered and enabled to make more adaptive choices for ourselves when triggered. It takes practice, for sure, and a practice like the one that follows—while it may seem very elementary—can help us break it down into more manageable chunks.

In this expressive arts practice, we invite you to go back to however you may have written out or listed your Dissociative Profile. Although some of these words may be helpful in facilitating understanding, words are often not the best fit at the level of the body. Take out a set of highlighters, colored pencils, markers, or any other drawing instrument that is color-coded, and start corresponding the words in the left-hand or trigger columns with colors. So for instance, when you read about getting yelled at by your boss, what color does that feel like? If a color doesn't seem to come up, is there a symbol that goes along with it, like a hammer? Perhaps you draw the hammer in the margins next to your Dissociative Profile. The color and the symbol may resonate, so perhaps you make your hammer red! And then finally, notice what it feels like in the body or where you experience the feeling of being yelled at in your body. Is it in your head? In your physical heart? If you are aware of the location or overall body sensation, note those.

After you've been able to color, symbol, and cue your stressors or triggers, go over to the right-hand column and engage in a similar practice. Are there any colors that go along with these experiences of relief or connection? Symbols? Body locations?

As you continue to track this information on your Dissociative Profile, stay aware of how it might show up in your daily life. When you start to feel a sense that a hammer is hitting you in your head, or a red wave of tension rise up in your chest—even before you recognize what might be bothering you or any of your parts—practice taking grounding or coping skill action in that moment to help you stay present. The fullness of the trigger may not even materialize, yet if it does, you will teach yourself over time to meet it with a greater sense of centering and presence.

══QUESTIONS TO ASK MY THERAPIST OR PSYCHIATRIST══

- Do you see dissociation as a phenomenon that happens on a continuum, or is there another explanation you like to use?
- How important is engaging in skills and strategies between our sessions?
- What kind of plan will we develop to help me/us manage affect and intensity between sessions?
- What are your feelings on the Window of Tolerance model? Do you think there are others that better account for dissociative experiences?

Below is a blank wheel of tolerance template you can use for your own mapping exercises.

Wheel of Tolerance

FIGHT
Hit, scream, brace, abuse, lash out, be sarcastic, dark humor, bully, dominate . . .

FLIGHT
Run, hide, "spin," fidget/stim, daydream, imagine, books/films, rationalize, dissociate . . .

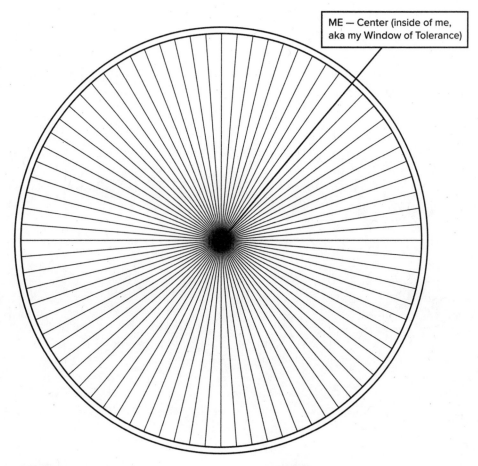

ME — Center (inside of me, aka my Window of Tolerance)

FREEZE
Dissociate, collapse, tonic immobility, catatonia, stuck, lose word/orientation/time/vision, faint . . .

FAWN
Please, appease, pledge, placate, submissive, succumb, obey . . .

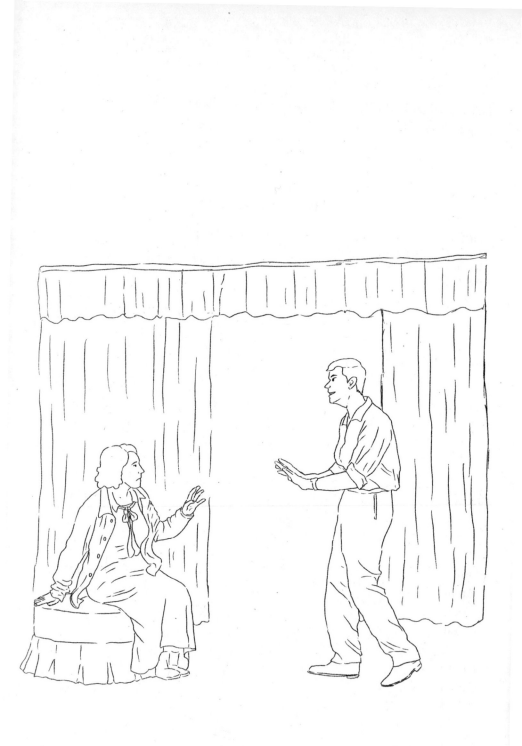

Options for Treatment and Healing

To heal is to touch with love that
which we previously touched with fear.
—STEPHEN LEVINE

Many definitions abound in trauma-focused circles on what constitutes healing. One of my favorite insights is from the teaching of Dr. Francine Shapiro, creator of EMDR Therapy. In speaking on the transformative power of EMDR Therapy, she explained that the purpose of EMDR is to help people live a more adaptive life.[1] What *adaptive* means can vary from person to person (and system to system). As we unpacked in chapter 1, the meaning of *adaptive* can change over time and depending on context. Such an open-ended definition of healing that allows for variance and change can be crucial for people struggling with dissociation, especially those diagnosed with a dissociative disorder. It's important that we not feel so boxed in, especially by institutions and approaches to therapy that may codify or manualize what healing *ought* to look like. . . .

The definition of healing that opens this chapter is from Dr. Shapiro's own mindfulness meditation teacher, the late Dr. Stephen Levine. Levine, known for his work with the chronically ill and those who are dying, brings a more poetic feel to our discussion. And even here, there is no set clinical definition on what healing ought to look like, other than inviting us to move from a place of fear to a place of love. This chapter explores how our various contributors have been able to make this shift in their healing journey. Some are still very actively in the process of making the shift, and others realize that healing will always come in layers unfolding through the seasons of life. One of our contributors, a woman with DID named BeeJay, summarizes the content of this chapter so powerfully, proclaiming, "Dissociation saved our lives. We may just need some help getting them back again."

We will present common themes that showed up in how our contributors have been able to engage a healing path and at least begin the process of getting their lives back. Many contributors actively speak from a state of living their lives to the fullest, from a place of thriving. The most pertinent theme that arose in examining responses to the question, "What, if anything, has been most effective for you so far in your process of healing?" is that no singular method did it. For all of our contributors, there is crediting of a combination of factors in their process. The chapter begins with some reflections on how an integration of approaches, both within the realm of professional psychotherapy and through other healing arts, worked for many of our contributors. A variety of contributors singled out a specific modality or approach that seemed to be a game changer for them, and the section that follows will look at several of these strategies as singular entities. Those strategies include EMDR Therapy, Somatic and Expressive Modalities, Traditional Addiction Treatment and 12-Step Modalities, Text-Based Therapy, Psychedelics and Plant Medicine, Yoga and Energy Modalities, Spiritual Direction, and Shamanic and Indigenous Approaches. Even in the individual sections, you will see how the need for healthy integration of approaches is still highlighted by our contributors.

Then, we present a Cautionary Tales section featuring reflections on what several contributors did not find helpful about certain therapeutic approaches. More of this content, directed at therapists, appears in our special Appendix written for clinicians and therapists. The chapter concludes with a section about the relational process of therapy and asks us to consider if *how* a therapist or healing arts practitioner operates is just as important—if not more important—than *what* they do in a session.

The Integration of Approaches

The International Society for the Study of Trauma and Dissociation (ISSTD) published treatment guidelines for both adults and adolescents dealing with dissociative disorders in 2011. These can be viewed online at no charge to you, and we provide the link in the Recommended Reading and Resources section. My assessment summary of these guidelines is that prudence within a trauma- and dissociation-informed model of care is vital, regardless of the specific therapy being used. One of our professional contributors, Dr. Deborah Korn, sheds some light on how she brings the spirit of these guidelines to life in her practice. Dr. Korn reports using a phase-oriented approach to treatment that is the standard throughout much of the trauma care being done in the world today. Originally developed by Pierre Janet himself in 1889, a phase-oriented approach to treatment follows this general flow:[2]

- Phase 1: Stabilization, symptom-oriented treatment, and preparation for liquidation (or elimination) of traumatic memories

- Phase 2: Identification, exploration, and modification (or shifting) of traumatic memories

- Phase 3: Relapse prevention, relief of residual symptoms, personality reintegration or addressing treatment goals around healing of ego states, and rehabilitation or transition to a healthier life

The phase model is applicable across theoretical orientations and specific modalities. According to Dr. Korn, no modality that we cover in this chapter is effective if you don't have a trauma- and dissociation-informed framework.

Relating specifically to working with DID and people with very defined parts, Dr. Korn sees herself as constantly doing group therapy with the presenting client. She is always working toward increasing someone's co-consciousness and to bring parts into communication, observing that "People need help with scooping up and then stitching together the components of experience." Dr. Korn maintains that the therapeutic relationship is *everything* in terms of creating a safe container for the work between the provider and their client. This relational container is essential for undoing the aloneness, and offering co-regulation that allows people to be courageous enough to approach the material that's been unapproachable.

For Holli Ellis, the signs of healing in her own life can show up when she is least expecting them. She will notice that she's able to wear a tighter shirt out in public and not be concerned that men are objectifying her. She can interact and smile with another parent; she can now be part of a collective or group and experience genuine connection. For Holli, the disease or illness model was a helpful starting point in addressing her eating disorder as a triage of sorts. But then she had to step back and look at the whole healing picture. While maintaining a connection to the literature of 12-step programs, she then began doing EMDR Therapy, which she initially judged as "the hokiest thing ever." Although the EMDR seemed to shift her to a different place, it never quite gave her the sense of peace or calm she was looking for. Adding yoga to her healing repertoire, which was also recommended by a therapist, "spoke to my soul and finally helped me to connect my soul and body."

Alicia Hann's journey to recovery began through multiple engagements of treatment for her eating disorder. Yet it wasn't until the last treatment episode that the team even began to explore trauma. She assessed previous experiences to be fundamentally unsuccessful because the trauma was not even touched. To attain meaningful recovery, Alicia began engaging in EMDR Therapy and has found the practice of Dancing Mindfulness helpful. And by approaching dance through a meditative, noncompetitive lens instead of a performance lens, Alicia has been able to work again as a professional dancer. Other practical strategies that Alicia enrolls in her healing include limiting her intake of alcohol, and distancing herself from certain family members.

Rebecca's description of her healing experiences in therapy also speaks to the power of integration. Prior to working with her current therapist, whom she first met in 2014, Rebecca reports only being exposed to cognitive behavioral therapy (CBT). Rebecca credits her current therapist's ability to be able to switch gears with modalities in helping her reach her goals, whereas in the past other therapists criticized her for needing to be more fluid. She engages in EMDR Therapy (with tappers or buzzers), EFT tapping, neurolinguistic programming (NLP), and parts work (using the Fraser's Table movie screen technique) with her therapist. She also describes her somatic practices of yoga, meditation, free-flowing dance, and chanting as supportive to her healing. Rebecca says that she remains on a small dose of a psychotropic medication (an antidepressant) but it's been significantly tapered down over the years.

Alexis also credits her therapist's ability to follow where she leads, reflecting, "Sometimes the parts come out and she lets them talk about what they want to talk about." Her current therapist uses a combination of dialectical behavior therapy (DBT) and mindfulness, together with a lot of expressive arts therapy and writing. She began working with an equine therapist several years ago, which is especially helpful to one of her younger parts.

Christy Dunn, a therapist with DID, credits a support group that she participates in for therapists with DID as crucial and life-changing. She says, "I was looking for this when I was first diagnosed with a dissociative disorder and was unable to find one." Christy reports working with a helpful, exceptional, very attuned, and non-controlling therapist—which is needed after she reported experiencing multiple therapy violations and boundary crossings from a previous therapist. Christy, who has been in therapy on and off for nearly ten years, said that art was the first natural healing practice that she stumbled onto in her home when she was two to three years old. She reflects, "Art was there to express pain without getting caught," and it was divorced enough from her plain reality to be safe.

Jaime Pollack attests that "anything not talking" was most successful in her healing journey. The biggest initial breakthroughs came from expressive arts therapy, play therapy, sand tray work, and writing. She also reported that some hypnosis and guided imagery were initially helpful to create internal structures that were more workable and allowed for a greater sense of containment. Jaime then proceeded to engage in EMDR Therapy, which she felt really took her healing to the next level, but only because Jaime was already well-connected to her system and her therapist took time to "get to know who the players were." In contrast, Jaime feels that a previous experience with EMDR Therapy was unsuccessful because the therapist did not have this awareness of Jaime's system (despite claiming she was a DID expert) and constantly referenced a textbook.

Jackson, the African American veteran we first met in chapter 1, has lived such an interesting and multifaceted life, it is little wonder that his healing brings in a combination of influences and perspectives. In his personal healing journey, he credits the impact of mindfulness and meditation practice, recognizing the value in "allowing the mind to flow from time to time and realizing you can bring it back." As noted in other chapters, Jackson finds that reading on trauma, especially the impact of trauma on society, and noticing how it applies to him is important. In addition to the archetypal wisdom he draws upon from Native American and African folklore, he also credits comedians as important members of his healing circle. Says Jackson, "Once you get people laughing, you open them up to thinking."

In addition to getting the professional treatment he needed, which started with a correct diagnosis of a dissociative disorder, John Fugett also emphasizes the importance of writing poetry and reading literature in his healing journey. He specifically credits Portuguese writer Fernando Pessoa, who wrote in the language of parts, as healing for him. All of these literary practices, he says, open up a part of him: "I need to be able to say these things."

In reflecting on a variety of spiritual practices that have helped her to heal (yoga, mantra meditation, energy work, loving connections with therapists), Susan Pease Banitt believes that they've assisted her in answering a core question: "What is the most healing environment for me to be in?" Both of our contributors named Paula also share keen summary insights. For Paula, "The things I fear the most are some of the things I embrace the most now: EMDR, reiki, Progressive Counting, sitting in those negative experiences that fueled the addictive behaviors." And for Paula S., "Therapy, specifically EMDR in combination with somatic therapy. Dance, music, massage, meeting some amazing people and being able to connect to them."

For Jacqueline Lucas, "EMDR helped me with quite a few things, yet in reflecting back on my healing it's also important to point out the reparative experiences that negated the not so great experiences. For example, having wonderful experiences with men who were kind, nurturing, and loving. I don't think men realize the power that they have to affect positive experiences of all kinds for female survivors." Danyale Weems connects to another form of experience in her healing: "When I read, I have a two-brain system: I can appreciate it for my clients and also how it applies to me. In addition to therapy, reading the stories of lived experience of people like Glennon Doyle and Brené Brown is helpful to me." And one of our anonymous contributors sums up her process as, "My healing has been a combination of a whole hell of a lot of work. I don't think there's ever going to be a magic bullet that I've seen with other people in terms of my healing."

Specific Modalities
EMDR Therapy

Because I am a public figure in the EMDR community, I recognize that many of the contributors who came forward to be interviewed found me through my work in EMDR Therapy. The fact that a high volume of contributors report exposure to EMDR Therapy is not necessarily an endorsement for the therapy as being superior to other modalities listed here. However, since we have so much lived experience shared about EMDR Therapy among the contributors, let's embrace it as a chance to learn about how this modality can work and what precautions may need to be taken. Two of our contributors reported that EMDR Therapy was not effective for them, and one spoke extensively about its mixed effectiveness. Extended sharing on these matters appears in the section to follow on Cautionary Tales.

EMDR stands for Eye Movement Desensitization and Reprocessing. The therapy, first published in a peer-reviewed journal in 1989, was formally discovered by Dr. Francine Shapiro. A cancer survivor highly interested in the intricacies of mind–body medicine, especially mindfulness meditation, Shapiro stumbled onto the mechanism of bilateral stimulation (back-and-forth motion) by taking a walk in the park. She noticed that as she entertained certain disturbing thoughts that emerged rather spontaneously, her eyes began to move back and forth. When she sat down and continued to engage in this process deliberately, she observed a lessening in disturbance about the intensity and validity of those thoughts. Following her initial trial-and-error experimentation, EMDR Therapy was developed and is now one of the most recognized treatments in the world for PTSD and other trauma-related disorders. The World Health Organization currently lists EMDR Therapy (along with CBT) as one of its two preferred methods in the treatment of PTSD.[3]

My personal therapist, Elizabeth Davis, who has also received EMDR Therapy, believes that it is the quickest way to bring about relief, especially if the therapist is attuned to working with parts. Following up on the previous section, which detailed Jaime Pollack's experiences with EMDR Therapy, Elizabeth believes that if one has DID or a dissociative disorder, getting an EMDR therapist comfortable with parts work and dissociation is important. As a personal and professional reflection on this insight, I am often asked if EMDR Therapy is effective for people with dissociative disorders. While I work vehemently to dispel this myth that EMDR Therapy is off-limits for dissociative disorders, I also recognize that if a person with a dissociative disorder is going to attempt EMDR Therapy, they must do it with a therapist who is unafraid of dissociation and skillful in navigating its manifestations.

Thomas Zimmerman, now an EMDR trainer and thought leader himself, began his journey with EMDR Therapy as a client. Thomas's primary traumatic experience was spiritual in nature, surviving years of cutting himself off from his very real human nature through engagement in practices he describes as Catholic mysticism. He engaged in a high degree of scrupulosity or rigidity in his religious practices during this time in his young adult life, often sleeping on hard surfaces to attain what he perceived as a higher degree of purification. Of these experiences, Thomas reports, "I felt like I was in the apartment adjacent to God but never in my body." Prior to his EMDR Therapy engagement, Thomas was already writing quite a bit and reports that having close, attuned, embodied friends who acted as mirrors for him was important. His EMDR therapist wisely knew they couldn't work on his spiritual trauma first as that was his hardest struggle, so they began by working on school and community violence he was exposed to in middle school, and abuse by his stepfather. Following this work, Thomas reports having enough adaptive information in place that the spiritual trauma work did not feel as big as it would have had they started there.

For Sandra Johnson, who is both an EMDR Therapy client and EMDR therapist, not being scared of dissociation within EMDR and letting each part be what that part needs to be is crucial. She contends, "The therapist has to have a much higher level of openness and lack of expectation about things happening." For Sandra, this is the key to doing good EMDR Therapy in general, not just doing good EMDR Therapy with multiplicity. Sandra's connection to what she describes as a skillful, human, and compassionate therapist is important. She reflects, "He never made me feel like anything was wrong with me, but he was also very good about holding boundaries even though every single part of me tested him. He went out and learned what he needed to learn and never put me into a stereotype."

Somatic and Expressive Modalities

Dr. Kellie Kirksey reports connecting with expressive practices like writing, sound healing, and dance from a young age. Kellie, who describes dance as her "critical medicine," believes that she would have ended up with a serious addiction if she didn't have these tools early in her life. For Erin, embodiment practices like yoga and the expressive arts helped her to heal the most. She reflects, "Those allowed for the embracing of healing as a whole and as a process. And I was able to see how everything flowed and connected to everything else." Erin recalls that in her youth she was exposed to many expressive modalities like writing, theater, playing music, and dancing. She also rode horses. In her estimation, she was not using any of these practices directly for her healing, yet "by proxy they helped me to survive." Because these practices came with a high degree of vulnerability for her, Erin notes that having a therapist meet her where she was at and provide some necessary psychoeducation about the brain was what allowed her to approach them in earnest. With candor, Erin explained, "I needed the foreplay of CBT and psychoeducation for sure."

Other practices that contributors named in the somatic realm include the trauma scholar Dr. Janina Fisher's approach to Internal Family Systems (IFS). Fisher is a trainer in Sensorimotor Psychotherapy (developed by Dr. Pat Ogden) and for the participant who named her, Fisher's somatic applications of IFS are innovative and helpful. Also named by a contributor is the closely related Somatic Experiencing, developed by Dr. Peter Levine. For sunnEe hope, who named Somatic Experiencing, specific practices like pendulation—or navigating in and out of the window of tolerance—are helpful, as is the responsive presence of her Somatic Experiencing Practitioner (SEP).

Traditional Addiction Treatment and 12-Step Modalities

Adam O'Brien, my collaborator on the Addiction as Dissociation model, began his recovery journey in a rehab center twelve years ago. In rehab he learned that the help was there, but that experience was devoid of the love. Through self-help approaches like the 12 steps and then later engaging in many of his own explorations, he learned to connect with the love. In the full Addiction as Dissociation model we posit that traditional approaches like the 12 steps can still be useful for certain people, as long as they are being utilized within a trauma- and dissociation-informed framework of care, as guided by Janet's phases.

On her experience with 12-step recovery, Fiona recalls, "I experienced so many occasions of kindness at 12-step meetings and got really lucky with sponsorship. And it was one of the first places I really belonged. Yet I've also had horrible things happen there too—being sexually assaulted, getting robbed, having my story sold to a newspaper. So we have to be careful not to present the 12 steps and meetings in a Utopian way." If you are interested in exploring further adaptation on the 12-step model through a more trauma-informed lens, please consider checking out my own *Trauma and the 12 Steps: An Inclusive Guide to Enhancing Recovery*, referenced in the Recommended Reading and Resources section.

For Megan, attending a treatment center to address her alcohol use disorder was vital to her recovery process. Although the center she went to incorporated some components of a 12-step model, she no longer attends meetings. She believes that being able to attend a treatment center with a program geared toward veterans and first responders was critical to her success. Megan reports that her therapist helped her identify the need for treatment and, together with Megan's best friend, found the right fit of a program for her. What is also impressive about Megan's therapist is that she initially felt she was not qualified to treat Megan for the DID. Yet because they were able to find an appropriate referral in the community, Megan's therapist got education and consultation. Megan is impressed by how her therapist, who is primarily an EMDR Therapist, was able to adapt.

Text-Based Therapy

One of the modalities that I did not expect to surface as significant, yet it did for one contributor, is text-based therapy on platforms like BetterHelp or Talkspace. Because this form of therapy is becoming more prevalent in our modern times, and because A.J., the contributor who identified it as helpful, offered a high degree of insight on *why,* we elected to address it as its own section. A.J., diagnosed with OSDD, has been in therapy on and off most of her life, and says that using the platform BetterHelp is more powerful than any traditional therapy she's received. Using the platform, she is able to send her therapist video messages in the moment, which seemed more beneficial than waiting to fit everything into a weekly session where she has a tendency to forget things. She also notes a tendency to forget things in between sessions, as dissociative amnesia can still pose a problem for her, reflecting, "There are many messages and video clips in the record with my current therapist that I have no memory of sending." A.J., who has worked with her therapist this way for three years, says, "I don't even need her to respond, yet being able to tell her things in a stream-of-consciousness manner has been the single most revealing thing ever for me."

The natural curiosity I had in interviewing A.J. about receiving therapy in this way related to therapeutic boundaries, and the potential for feeling rejection if the therapist doesn't respond as much as the client would like them to over this text platform. A.J. acknowledges that it can be hard for people to interpret boundaries as anything but rejection, so she advises that therapists working in this way set the boundaries immediately. Being transparent about expected response times, level of commitment, and having a safety plan in place if the client does not get a response right away are all important. As the client, get used to hearing a line like, "I am here for you in this capacity" from your therapist.

Psychedelics and Plant Medicine

There is a growing interest throughout trauma and addiction treatment on integrating psychedelics and other plant medicines into a person's healing experience. As a person in abstinence-based recovery I was initially skeptical about integrating highly psychoactive drugs into treatment, yet my perspective gradually broadened. First of all, the emerging clinical data on psychedelic treatment's effectiveness with a variety of mental health conditions simply cannot be ignored. Secondly, in speaking to many collaborators and friends on the utility of psychedelics and traditional plant medicines in healing, I was inspired to try out a psilocybin experience under the guidance of a Shamanic practitioner as part of my preparation for this book. I spoke with my own 12-step sponsor and therapist about it, and we all felt it was a good idea at this point in my healing journey to get at some additional layers that my previous healing work had not quite addressed. And I was not left disappointed.

Not only the psychedelic experience, but also the continued follow-up work with my Shamanic practitioner who skillfully guided me, have facilitated potent experiences in unraveling what I feel has rooted in my heart and soul from traumatic experiences and their fallout. Using the metaphor of the snake and the venom, I feel like previous therapeutic experience with EMDR Therapy and deeper yoga practice helped to get the venom out. Yet the psilocybin experience, combined with the Shamanic practitioner's skillful guidance, helped to get the dead roots from the fangs out of me. And in the process, my connection to what the theologian Pierre Teilhard de Chardin called "the breathing together of all things"[4] beautifully expanded.

The word *psychedelic* comes from a Greek root meaning "mind manifesting," and as a classification of drugs, they are considered hallucinogens that trigger non-ordinary states of consciousness. Mescaline, LSD, psilocybin, and DMT are the best known psychedelics, with related compounds like MDMA and ketamine also entering the discussion on therapeutic benefits. Ayahuasca, a combination of a psychedelic and an entheogen (a psychoactive substance that alters mood and perception), has also been discussed more fully in recent years, and the addiction specialist Dr. Gabor Maté recently promoted its use in his new documentary *The Wisdom of Trauma*.[5] Ayahuasca has traditionally been used in the ceremonial medicine of Indigenous peoples of the Amazon basin in South America. As with many issues covered in this book, there is so much material out there on the therapeutic use of psychedelics and related compounds, we encourage you to visit the Recommended Reading and Resources section in the back of the book if you wish to explore further to determine whether seeking out this type of treatment is right for you. In this section, we primarily focus on the wisdom of our contributors.

Tada Hozumi, who actively engages in psychedelic experiences, defines *psychedelic* as "the experience of swimming through a collective nervous system to see how it operates. *Psychedelic* is the difference between theoretical and being alive." For Melissa Parker, a therapist with DID who advocates for other therapists, a combination of therapy and MDMA treatment was her game changer. Although MDMA is widely known as the street drug Ecstasy and the center point of the rave scene, there is emerging evidence of its effectiveness in the treatment of PTSD,[6] although it is still widely banned throughout North America for official medical use.

Melissa, age forty-eight at the time of her interview, began taking MDMA around the age of thirty-three. She reports that it anchored her into the breath and it was the first thing that brought her into her body, allowing her to notice many things she previously hadn't. She ended up taking a lot of MDMA trips in the years to follow, never with the intention that it would be healing or therapeutic, yet that happened for her. She says, "I was able to look at every shitty thing in my life and acknowledge the hurt. I learned how to accept myself. I learned how to pull out little pieces of the trips and apply them to my daily care, and the care of my system. It comes down to being able to hold the pain."

Adam O'Brien's wisdom is featured throughout the book, and of course his embrace of innovative recovery paths also brought him to psychedelics. On his personal experience Adam shares, "I knew it was a dangerous game to play because addictions can take on various forms. When I did psychedelics under the care of a therapeutically minded guide, I realized that my previous use was from societal immaturity that didn't allow for healing. Psychedelics can help people to heal and to discover. They pushed my boundaries and limits and then brought me back to my body, where I traditionally dissociated because of my pain management issues."

Adam, who fully believes that Western frameworks lack the nuance to fully understand dissociation, also serves in a professional capacity by guiding his clients in a service called *psychedelic integration*. Adam assists people in taking what they receive during psychedelic or similar plant medicine experiences and weaving it into their psychotherapeutic work. Susan Pease Banitt, whose feelings about Western psychotherapy as limited are well-documented throughout this book, continues to notice that microdosing of psychedelics is becoming critical to helping many traumatized people experience the expansion of the soul. Melissa Parker is working to develop a nonprofit organization that will help survivors of trauma and those navigating life with dissociation to be able to access MDMA.

We will see the most growth and discussion in this area over the next several years. I am happy to see that people like Adam, Susan, and Melissa are on the front lines of creating a meaningful integration between use of these psychedelic experiences and other healing modalities. As Adam observed, addiction can take on many forms. When I see white people from North America heading to South America to engage in ayahuasca ceremonies multiple times a year, I do skeptically wonder if they might be missing the point. Can we become addicted to the experience of psychedelics and feel like we *need it* in order to connect to our larger sense of consciousness? According to Julian Jaramillo, his Shamanic teacher from the Chocó people of Ecuador does not emphasize constant use, "just a few times, to help you see."

Michael Pollan, in his landmark book *This Is Your Mind on Plants,* contends that people in the West have much to learn from Indigenous cultures who have made use of psychedelics like mescaline and ayahuasca in sacred healing. He notes, "As a rule, the substances are never used casually, but always with intention and surrounded by ritual and under the watchful eye of experienced elders." There is recognition by Pollan and those he consulted for the book that plant medicine can tap into powerful emotions and energies that can "get out of control if they are not managed with care."[7]

Like any therapeutic experience discussed in this book, I advise you to do your homework if psychedelics or similar experiences are calling to you. Especially because issues around legality can be precarious depending on where you live in the world, connecting with a word-of-mouth network to find an ideal guide is likely better than just idly searching online. As I reflect on my own experience, the psilocybin treatment would have fallen flat without having such a wise guide whom I trusted based on previous work I did with her in other modalities. Moreover, having other resources for healing around me, both before and after the psychedelic experience, allowed so many connections and linkages to be made. I truly feel like my recovery has entered new territory.

Yoga and Energy Modalities

We've elected to cover yoga here rather than earlier, when we spoke about somatic modalities. Even though yoga emerged many times in the question asked about grounding (see chapter 3), yoga specific to deeper healing practices better falls into the realm of energetic healing, not just a simple somatic practice. We as human beings are energetic creatures. If you are not embracing of this idea, I challenge you to go ahead and rub your hands together right now. Build up some friction and heat. Then, gently pull the hands apart. What are you feeling or noticing? Then let yourself slowly draw the hands back together but do not let them touch. What are you noticing now?

If the simple answer that came up for you was heat or sensation, know that this is energy. Energy is all around us. Even if it's a stretch for you to see the human body as an energetic vehicle, have you ever referred to something (or someone) as having a negative energy? Or a positive energy? Have you ever referred to yourself as being depleted of energy? Another way to think of energy is *life force*. And unhealed trauma can drain us of life force. As it relates to dissociation, many of us with parts, whether we switch often or not, describe an experience of feeling drained of energy when one of our parts might demand more time and attention of us than usual. And as The Garden System described in chapter 4, their frequent switching can lead to energetic chaos in the body, making essential the need for grounding and skills that help to realign their energetic balance. For her, EFT (emotional freedom techniques) tapping, and engaging in the gentle back and forth "butterfly tap" on her upper arms, an EMDR-inspired technique, are helpful.

As first noted in chapter 3, several contributors named energetic practices like reiki or cranial sacral massage as essential to their grounding, and reiki came up several more times later in the interviews as being supportive of deeper healing practices. For one of our anonymous contributors with OSDD, "I never felt my feet on the ground until reiki." Interestingly, she told me this three times over the course of our ninety-minute interview. This is the same contributor who also credited being outside as vital to her overall well-being, commenting, "I am a person of disconnection and nature is fully a place of connection."

The complete practice of yoga is one that can facilitate a sense of energetic cleansing and balancing while also promoting deep connection. When I refer to the complete practice of yoga, I am referencing the full system, the Eight Limb practice that originated in India. For many in the West, the limbs of *asana* (poses) and *pranayama* (breath, or quite literally, the movement of the life force) are the only two associations. Classical yoga involves limbs dedicated to life ethics and the fundamentals of how to get to a meditative state. In the true spirit of *system,* one of my teachers from India would say that even if you are only practicing in one limb you are practicing in the others. Hence, the Western commercialization of yoga doesn't necessarily bother him because practicing something, even if it is poses and breath, can eventually lead you to the meditative heart of the practice. Our contributor Erin had this experience. She originally began practicing yoga as a fitness-based endeavor in a typical American studio to help her with running. Erin is now a certified yoga teacher who has traveled to India and is steeped in the meditative and cultural elements of the practice.

Malika, one of our contributors with complex trauma, has been on a serious healing journey the last ten years of her life. Malika has received both traditional talk therapy and EMDR Therapy in this endeavor. Although she grew up in India, her exposure to yoga did not fully happen until she was living in the United States, where she deepened her study through teacher training. Now living back in India and studying there, she offers us a very nuanced understanding of how the meditative elements of yoga can work together with psychological methods to help clear a path. Malika truly believes that healing is her *dharma,* or what she sees as her purpose for this life. In Malika's belief system, which is shared by many throughout the world, she came into this life carrying *samskaras,* or impressions, from the wounds of past lives. In her case, she believes that some nasty adults took advantage of her nature, which makes her wonder if kids who are spiritually inclined tend to get abused more, so their *samskaras* from past lifetimes can be revealed, providing opportunities to heal in this lifetime.

Malika recalls that when her healing began, it initially felt too intense. Sometimes it can still feel too intense for her, and in those moments reminding herself that "healing is my *dharma*" can be helpful. When she is triggered or notices other intensity, she literally feels heat rising in her body. And she has learned this is a signal that the *samskaras* are being burned. Three principles of yoga help her ride out this intensity until the energy clears: *tapas* (letting the heat work on you), *svadhyaya* (self-study or examination), and *Ishvara Pranidhana* (surrender to God or something greater than her). Malika says that even though she learned these principles prior to the COVID-19 pandemic, the new reality of living in the pandemic gave her more opportunities to practice. She reflects, "When these three aspects of kriya yoga come into your life, you are burning the seeds; the impressions. You are no longer living on survival tactics."

Spiritual Direction

We recognize that if you do not see yourself as a religious or spiritual person, or if abuse in this realm was part of your story, what Malika has to share about yoga might feel inaccessible. Please be reminded that you do not have to force all of the practices in this book to be a good fit for you. We are simply sharing what has worked for others in their journey and you can decide if it's something that might resonate for you.

Two of our contributors mentioned spiritual direction from a progressive Christian perspective as being necessary to their healing process. Spiritual direction is just what the name suggests—work done in individual or group settings that is not therapeutic in nature, yet meant to be supportive of one's spiritual journey. One does not have to be a licensed minister or clerical professional to offer spiritual direction, nor do they have to specifically practice pastoral counseling. As with many healing arts, the quality and training of spiritual directors can vary, so you are also advised to do your homework if seeking out a spiritual director feels like a good fit for you. Visiting the home page of Spiritual Directors International is a good start (a link is provided in the Recommended Reading and Resources section).

Kylie, who identifies as a survivor of sexual and spiritual abuse, has been in spiritual direction for the past ten years. She describes the work as transformational to her healing. Kylie explains,

> My spiritual director brings my faith into my life in terms of guidance. She would say it's listening to the spirit, listening to God talk through her. This is so powerful because it's an experience I have of God and the Divine that is happening in real time. Being challenged in a healthy way in the context of a relationship. You're not being told what to do. I've experienced more healing and faster dealing in spiritual direction than in therapy. I see it as the power of the Holy Spirit.

For Dianne Harper, whom we met in chapter 4 as she offered her experience with parts integration, a brief stint attending seminary eventually led her to a program for offering spiritual direction to others. In her training program, she experienced many opportunities to do her own work through Jungian archetypes, which combined nicely with her existing practice of Soul Collage (a creative modality for introspection). As someone who's explored many different paths to spirituality, these methods in combination strike Dianne as more fluid and enriching for her at this stage in her life, instead of constantly working on family of origin issues in traditional therapy. She clarifies that while she still sees a traditional therapist once a month, they are not directly dealing with the effects of the abuse as they did extensively in the past, even if they may still find the need to touch on family of origin issues.

Shamanic and Indigenous Approaches

In her continued commentary on Western psychotherapy, author and contributor Susan Pease Banitt declares, "The problem with Western medicine is that it is inherently dissociative. That comes out of the Inquisition, when we divorced our intellect from our Indigenous [or organic] natures." Even if you don't connect with Susan's exact expression of her experience, we hope that this idea of Eurocentric medicine and psychology not having all of the answers (and perhaps creating many of the problems) is well-established in this book. In chapter 3 we began examining how some of our contributors are connecting to Native and Indigenous practice as a more organic and holistic experience of healing. While there are a variety of ceremonies and traditions that could fall under the purview of this section, we are focusing on the practice of sweat lodge *(Inipi)* since it came up the most for our contributors. And during my own preparation for this book, I had a chance to participate in healing rituals with a Blackfeet community and a group of mostly white veterans around the practice of sweat.

Roger Vielle, a Blackfeet elder who we first met in the introduction, explains that in modern times the Sioux Nation really began working with the principle of sweat—the ritual blending of fire, water, and healing herbs—to prepare men for going to war and to transition them back into their home life upon returning from war. In getting to know Roger, I've learned about the mythology he was taught as a Blackfeet elder for how sweat originated as a healing practice. If you have the privilege and opportunity one day of engaging in an authentic sweat lodge experience, I encourage you to ask the person guiding you how their nation or tribe sees the healing practice of sweat from a cultural or mythological standpoint. While they may or may not be willing to share it with a non-Native individual, if they are willing to share the origins with you, be open to their teachings on how these origin stories might inspire your healing journey today. For Roger, sweats are a form of good medicine, and when he offers them, he doesn't see it as *him*. It is the *Creator*. To him, as a veteran who works with other veterans, it would be ideal if people who return ·from war have somewhere they can go in the transition so they don't bring trauma from war into their homes. And it's equally essential for their spouses and families to receive this support too.

Although I was greatly intrigued listening to people as they discussed their experiences with sweat lodges over the years and through early interviews, I got very excited to learn more when I met Brandon Spangler. Brandon, a Marine veteran in long-term recovery from heroin and methamphetamine addiction, is passionate about the practice of sweat and facilitating experiences for other veterans. Brandon is also a licensed clinician in the state of Montana and sees how therapeutic practices including EMDR Therapy can fuse naturally with the practice of sweat. Brandon reflects,

> In most of the sweats I've done you literally call yourself back from having a traumatic experience. I think that's a big one. It's recognizing that something is missing or something has been distorted. There are also different sweat rituals focused on different things. And I've had a chance to process a lot of my

childhood stuff in there too. In therapy, people can get really "heady," intellec-
tualize what's happening. But when you're really, really, really hot, yeah, the
bullshit gets pushed aside.

For TaNiya, our contributor we met in chapter 2 who reported both a
DID and a Borderline Personality Disorder diagnosis, everything in the Shamanic realm needs to be taken more seriously by therapists in the Western
mainstream. Speaking to the connection with MDMA we brought up in a
previous section, TaNiya noticed she was starting to process even before she
fully entered addiction recovery by taking Ecstasy at raves. Then, her work
with a Shamanic practitioner over the last five years allowed her to connect
even more material, especially trauma that is intergenerational in nature. She
reflects, "For me, parts work and Shamanism both work for me because they
are the same thing—healing the fragmented stuff."

Cautionary Tales

The most consistent cautionary tale that appeared throughout the interviews
was participants' belief that their therapists did not know what they were
doing, or that the participants seemed to be "too much" for the therapists
they were seeing. Insights on what therapists can do to become more aware
of facilitating a quality working relationship appear in our first Appendix, for
clinicians and therapists. Remember that it is not the job of a therapist or
other healing professional to be your best friend or your replacement parent.
Yet if you do not feel a sufficient level of comfort and safety with them, any
technique or approach they try with you will likely fall flat. So at any time
during your healing journey if you are not feeling the connection you believe
you need to be experiencing, address this with them. See what solutions they
might offer. If you are still not feeling great about what they offer to repair any
breaches in the relationship, please know that you are empowered to look
elsewhere. Even if you are a non-therapist reading this book, I still encourage
you to check out the Appendix written for clinicians and therapists so you
can get a better sense of what our contributors identified as important to their
healing experience.

In the interviews, several techniques or approaches were specifically
flagged by contributors as problematic. Destiny Aspen Mowadeng, whose
insights appear throughout the book, notes that cognitive behavioral therapy
(CBT) and dialectical behavior therapy (DBT) were both unhelpful for her.
She found them "triggering, dismissive, and invalidating," and also found that

much of the terminology used in both therapies ignored the experiences of disabled people. Ultimately, she found that working with a trauma coach was most helpful to her, instructing her in the basics of trauma-informed mindfulness and getting some of the psychoeducation that she needed. I believe that both CBT and DBT can have their place in someone's healing. Yet in and of themselves, they will likely be insufficient for working with intense dissociation, especially in the hands of an unskilled therapist. Destiny recognizes that the therapist she had at the time could have been the culprit for why her experiences with these therapies were so negative.

Two of our contributors, one with OSDD and one with DID, said quite definitively that EMDR Therapy did not work for them even though their therapists were initially optimistic. Both seemed to indicate that the level of flashback during the EMDR process was too intense for them, and when they retreated into other skills to address the flashbacks, they ultimately found the other skills to be more meaningful to their help overall.

Perhaps the greatest examination I can do on why EMDR Therapy may not be a good fit for someone who dissociates significantly came by interviewing one of my former clients who came forward as a contributor. And she rightfully called me out on a few things!

Crystal stopped all therapy about four years prior to engaging in this interview. As a survivor of complex trauma due to various forms of abuse, Crystal was in and out of medical and mental health systems for years, diagnosed with everything but a dissociative disorder, and her trauma was rarely addressed. Crystal said that the happiest, healthiest time in her adult life was when she was able to ride her horse competitively, but a chronic medical condition prohibited her riding several years ago. In addition to dealing with that grief, Crystal identified that she lost her best coping skill. Even though she still goes to visit her horse, the grief is sometimes unbearable.

Crystal's psychiatrist referred her to me primarily for EMDR Therapy. We started there, and I eventually brought in more expressive arts therapy interventions. Looking back on her experience with therapy, she identifies that the expressive arts therapy—which included writing, collage work with glass, and dance—was the most helpful. These expressive interventions combined with just being able to talk and be heard really made an impression.

Crystal remembers that sometimes EMDR Therapy was useful, yet many times it just gave her more of a reason to dissociate. EMDR is known for being an extremely nonverbal and nondirective therapy. In EMDR Therapy you can do a lot with very little detail or actual narrative content about a traumatic event. We don't ask many questions of people about the traumatic incidents themselves, which is what many find appealing about the therapy. The flip side is that EMDR Therapy does encourage you to feel a great deal of emotion, body sensation, and affect that you may have kept yourself from feeling at the time of the experience. Letting yourself notice these things or "go with them" as we say in EMDR Therapy, as the therapist applies alternating eye movements, taps, or audio tones, is how this therapy can work so quickly to shift how memories are stored at the level of the brain. The entire process, guided by the EMDR Therapist yet directed by the client, is designed to engage shifts from the limbic brain to the neocortex, which is more efficient in long-term storage.

We generally do not talk much in EMDR Therapy and for Crystal, this was a big part of the problem. She reflected, "You would say *go with that*. Go where? I wanted more structure." She also said that sometimes she needed to just talk and receive validation from me, when I would seem too eager to keep the EMDR Therapy process going. In looking back on Crystal's case, I agree with her assessment. Sometimes EMDR Therapists can feel such a sense of, "I can help them get to the root of this and clear it so they can live a more adaptive life." We can lose sight of the essential humanity that good therapy requires. I believe I was so determined to help Crystal be relieved of her core trauma's pain, I didn't pay attention to everything else as much as I could have.

When clients share experiences about EMDR Therapy not working for them, there are some cases where I truly believe it's not the right fit. Crystal believes, as do I, that therapists have to be proficient in many modalities so that they can go with a flow if the modality they are originally placing the most faith in does not seem to work. Taking such an approach is essential for quality work through a dissociation-informed lens. As we've brought up many times in this book, linear rigidity or strict adherence to any one method is not the best strategy. Since dissociative minds are known for their fluidity and yes, sometimes a great deal of unpredictability, it's important to find a therapist or healing professional who will match this energy.

The Relational Process of Therapy and Healing Arts

Amy Wagner has seen a thought leader in the EMDR community for twelve years as her personal therapist; yet in that time they've actually done very little EMDR Therapy. Amy states that what worked best was her therapist's uncanny ability to challenge and be real with her. The therapeutic relationship is paramount to Amy, and she defines secure attachment within the therapeutic relationship as "really feeling seen and heard, and learning to tolerate that building intimacy is a process."

For several other contributors, being seen and heard was also a necessary base for therapy to be meaningful. Blaise offers, "It's a combination, but therapy is the biggest thing that's helped me work through my issues. My therapist is someone who can read what I need: tough love (the first responder in me) and unconditional support (being heard)." Michelle Kahl, a former paramedic crew chief now working as a trauma therapist, believes the most important thing for her was to feel validated, for her story to be believed. She said, "Something about his [my therapist's] demeanor gave me a chance, showed me that he really cared, he believed me and I felt like I had a chance at living and working through my trauma." Cheryl also sings the praises of her current therapist, maintaining that he changed her life. She notes, "He asks a lot of questions, is good at grounding me, and he really knows what he's doing." Kathleen explains that the relational foundation set by her therapist included just getting to know her, talking about anything—even politics and religion—without getting into an argument. For Kathleen, this relational foundation is what set the stage for her to be open to EMDR Therapy, which she experienced as something quite "magical."

Heather (LS) Scarboro+, themselves a therapist with DID, does not recognize a specific modality as being the most helpful in their journey, more so a combination of factors that have led to good therapy:

validation from therapist + trust in the therapist + trust in the system =
trust in the process

Heather (LS+) says nothing shuts them down quite like hearing therapists tell parts to "hush." They remember being one of the first people with DID that one of their therapists treated, yet it made an impression that this therapist knew when it seemed appropriate to get out of the office and do something active with the younger parts. Once, they got some fish for the counseling center fish tank. They also recognized when Will, their four-year-old part, was activated, how playing the game Simon Says was needed.

Fiona, our contributor from the United Kingdom whose insights appear throughout the book, expresses, "In Eurocentric therapies, the burden is

unduly placed on the 'patient' to heal. We must acknowledge that dissociation exists because the world is a harsh, unkind place most of the time."
For Katharine, a therapist with DID who struggled with the stigma around
it for quite some time, knowing that there was a word for dissociation was
validating of her experiences. For her, it's imperative that a professional in
any modality be able to say, "'I'm so honored that you're willing to share
that with me,' and not look at me like I have three heads. The minute a professional puts off a vibe that they don't know what to do with me, I'm done
with them."

Perhaps you've been in therapy before or perhaps this is your first time.
Either way, if you are inspired to seek out professional help after reading this
chapter, consider reflecting on what has worked or not worked in the past,
and what you might need differently at this time in your life. If you are a first-
timer to therapy, what are some qualities of a therapist that our contributors
described that are most healing to you? And as a final note, please also consider that practices other than professional, Western psychotherapy might be
the best fit for you at this time. If you are feeling jaded by the experience of
therapy right now, especially if you've struggled with trauma and dissociation
and it's been invalidated, you are not alone.

Healing has happened since the dawn of time, for centuries before professional psychotherapy even came into existence. So while I still believe that
the innovations of our modern times can be useful to us on our path of recovery, however we may choose to define it, psychotherapy does not have the
market cornered on healing. Whatever path emerges for you that helps you
do the work—to embrace your humanity in all of its fullness and not further
dissociate from it—we encourage you to follow that path. And may this path
also be one that guides you in how to honor the humanity in others while also
being kind to yourself or your selves.

A turning point for Thomas Zimmerman, whose story we more fully
explored in this chapter, is when he went to the Catholic sacrament of confes-
sion with a ninety-year-old priest. The priest, concerned by Thomas's intense
scrutiny of himself, gently advised him, "Remember, God created you to be
human." And that began Thomas's journey away from the most destructive of
his dissociative tendencies into the fullness of his humanity.

As I've pored over my notes on these interviews, the priest's guidance is
one of the pieces of wisdom that resonated for me the most. Because even
though I believe, like Carl Jung, that there is something bigger and greater

out there that unites us all; even though I believe in the power of spiritual practice to heal . . . I've also learned that fully embracing my humanity is the most Divine practice of them all.

No separation, no pathologizing.

Rather, learning to delight in the fullness of who we are.

Touching our wounds, our story, and indeed our parts . . . with love.

EXPRESSIVE ARTS PRACTICE: WRITING YOUR OWN HEALING MYTHOLOGY

In this chapter we mentioned that many Indigenous nations and tribes have their own healing mythologies to explain how practices like sweat might work. Although I encourage you to seek out one of these stories from a Native elder themselves, you can also look up many online; or consider checking out the work of Chris Stark, a woman with DID who identifies as Ojibwe, Cherokee, and European, cited in the Recommended Reading and Resources section. In chapter 4 you read the story of Hanuman as told in Hindu mythology, and took in wisdom from Shaman Julian Jaramillo about the importance of working with the stories in his traditions. You've also had a chance to witness me geek out on some pieces of popular culture, especially movies that I hold most dear.

Drawing from any sources of inspiration that feel right for you, you are now invited to write your own healing mythology or story. You may consider consulting your parts map from chapter 4 to help you with some of the characterization, or your scene writing from chapter 5 to help with some of the plot points. The story does not have to be long, or you can make it as long as you wish. If someone was reading the story of your hero's journey, how would it flow?

Be as creative and as expressive as you wish! As with all of our practices, you can allow this one to unfold over a period of several days or weeks. If the story is still being written as your life is currently being lived and your healing is still in process, how can you conclude the story in a way that feels open-ended, maybe even using a line like *to be continued* . . . ?

If it feels organic to bring in other expressive forms like drawing, photographs, filmmaking, songs/putting together a playlist, or dance, please follow those promptings and let it flow!

◄◄QUESTIONS TO ASK MY THERAPIST OR PSYCHIATRIST►►

- What is the main therapeutic modality that you presently use?

- Are you open to blending different therapeutic modalities?

- What are your feelings on bringing in practices like psyche-delic experiences or Indigenous healing arts to work alongside psychotherapy?

- If the main therapeutic modality you practice doesn't seem to be working for me, how do you approach making adjustments?

- How do you handle it if it seems like your clients are struggling with the therapy relationship? Are you open to having me say something if that feels like the case?

- What are some of the boundaries you need to set in working with people who are similar to me, or people you've treated with my diagnosis?

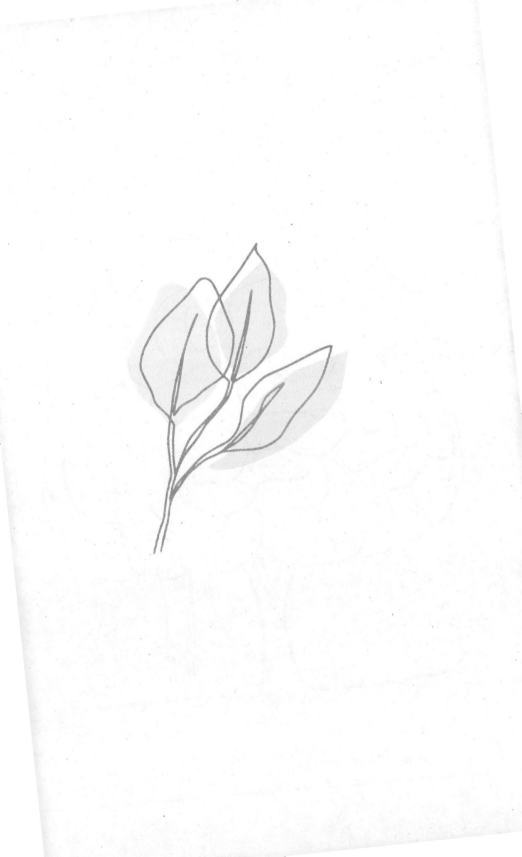

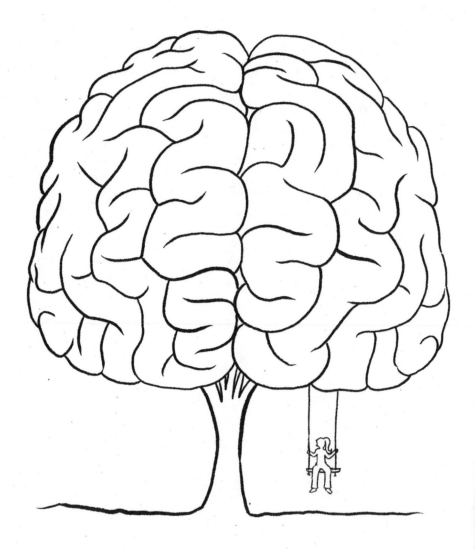

7

Removing the Stigma and Creating a New Narrative

I am absolutely uninterested in shame.
—ANNALYNNE MCCORD

"Setting the record straight" and "creating a new narrative" came up many times in interviews as the reason contributors wanted to participate in this book project. These sentiments rang strongest from our contributors who have dissociative disorders and also serve as clinical professionals. The myths and misconceptions about dissociation and dissociative disorders are abundant. Yet perhaps one of the greatest battles we've had to face, and are still facing, is this distorted belief that dissociation is not a real thing and that dissociative disorders, especially DID, are not real.

Katharine, one of our contributors who works as a therapist, said she regularly hears psychiatrists refer to DID as "bunk."

I wish I could say that this report is an outlier. I've heard it my entire clinical career, and sadly, it's still happening with great regularity.

One of my favorite responses I've heard to these now-common insults is from Olga Trujillo, a lawyer and advocate who has been out about their DID for quite some time. When a clinician told them, "I don't believe in DID," Olga responded, "I'm really glad you don't have to believe in it, and I don't have a choice because I have it. It's not a religion."

I've followed Olga's work for years and was delighted that they agreed to be interviewed as a contributor for this project. Olga's own memoir *The Sum of My Parts,* published in 2011, gives needed dimension to our humanizing of dissociative disorders. As a Latinx, native Spanish-speaking queer individual who was first diagnosed with DID when they were working as a lawyer for the U.S. Department of Justice, Olga's story has numerous layers. And their memoir also gives a detailed account of how long-term engagement in psychodynamic psychotherapy, together with their own exploration of mythology, helped facilitate their healing process. Olga says, "It is my passion to destigmatize DID."

They regularly give trainings for both clinical professionals and those in the legal system—judges, lawyers, and law enforcement personnel. Olga, who describes the American criminal and legal system as "inherently triggering" believes that if we continue to stay neutral about trauma, abuse, and dissociation, we are upholding the status quo. And this status quo mandates that survivors of trauma *prove* our stories in environments where lawyers are all too eager to exploit the impact of trauma. One of the long-term problems I've identified with the legal system—and Olga echoes this concern—is that if a survivor can't tell their story in a logical, linear manner, they are not believed. Because of how unhealed trauma is stored in the limbic brain—which does not operate on a rational, organized time scale—such a "keep your story straight" expectation is not realistic, at least until a survivor has been given what they need to process it. Moreover, linear conceptualization is not how dissociative minds work, or the type of dissociation responses that can overcome a person who is triggered may shut down any capacity for organized thinking. Hence, Olga will not do a "trauma-informed" training for the legal system without also covering dissociation and DID.

Olga recalls a story of a judge who once said DID was "poppycock," not understanding how someone can be so calm and composed one moment and so hysterical the next. When Olga shared this story, I was taken back to the moment of my second divorce (from the husband who filmed my dissociative episode), where I was activated and then actively dissociated through the proceedings. The judge asked me the value of my house and I could only vaguely comprehend hearing her speak, let alone be able to cogently answer her questions. She made the comment, "I remember what I paid for my house all the way back in 1978, how can you not remember?"

Here in this moment, calm and composed, I could have answered her question. But not when the reminders of abuse and toxicity in the marriage were dancing around me. I simply collapsed, and was so grateful that the judge was eventually able to see that what was happening with me was some type of abuse response. Olga said that they do see glimmers of hope in our legal system, with trauma-informed courts and trauma-informed legal advocacy surfacing with greater regularity. Yet there is still a long way to go with educating the general public, the legal system, and sadly, the clinical professions on the reality of dissociation and how it can manifest in people's lives. In Olga's view, we must continue to normalize trauma responses.

Many of our contributors are working to normalize the responses of trauma by coming out with their own stories. The depth and breadth of their sharing is what forms the heart of this book and I am grateful to them for it. Yet many of our contributors also have something to share on their fears about coming out publicly and how they'll be perceived. Several contributors noted, echoing my experience, that it feels easier to say you have PTSD because there is more acceptance around that diagnosis at a societal level. Yet introducing dissociation or a dissociative disorder into the mix can feel like navigating a minefield. How are people going to perceive me, especially if their only reference for anything "multiple" is a movie like *Sybil*? Olga says, "I am typical of someone with DID, but I am not stereotypical." And so many contributors came forward specifically to challenge the stereotypes and show that there are many ways to be dissociative and even have a dissociative disorder in the world.

There are many tasks to accomplish in this chapter as we discuss how to remove stigma around dissociation and dissociative disorders, and work toward creating a new narrative in the public forum. We will first establish what some of the myths, misconceptions, stereotypes, and controversies are around dissociation, specifically dissociative disorders. Then, we'll take a look at some of the problems with media portrayal surrounding dissociation. This section features an interview with a director who recently finished making a documentary that follows a woman with DID, and also provides commentary on media portrayal from some of our contributors. Then we conclude the chapter by having our contributors share their ideas for how we can dismantle stigma around mental health in general, specifically dissociation, and how we can empower ourselves to be self-advocating voices for change.

Myths, Misconceptions, Stereotypes, and Controversies

The main reason I did not begin the book by exploring these issues in any depth is because—quite frankly—I don't give them any credence. When I first began my graduate studies in clinical counseling (2003–2005), I was taught that "true DID is rare—there have only been 200 documented cases since the dawn of time." At my second major place of employment where I met my first DID client (to my knowledge anyway), clinical leadership discouraged me from "indulging" his belief that he had DID, insisting that he was attention-seeking or just psychotic. The way they advised me to treat that client never sat right with me, especially since so much came into focus just a few years prior when I was diagnosed with my own dissociative disorder. At that point I decided to personally deepen my study into working with dissociative disorders, especially within an EMDR context, and I haven't regretted the decision since.

We do feel it's important to cover what some of these major issues are so that you, the reader, are aware of them. Even if everything you've read about dissociative disorders has resonated for you so far, we are still living in a world that can be inhospitable to people like us. And depending on where you end up for clinical care, the reality may be equally brutal. As we will discuss at the end of the chapter, the decision is ultimately yours on how you might navigate these realities, especially if you decide to come out publicly about your dissociative mind.

In the article "Separating Fact from Fiction: An Empirical Examination of Six Myths about Dissociative Identity Disorder," Dr. Bethany Brand and colleagues identify and challenge the six most pervasive myths about DID.[1] The full scholarly article is available as an open access piece online, and you are encouraged to look it up if you'd like to read it in further depth. Here is a summary of myths they used peer-reviewed data to refute:

1 DID is a fad

2 DID is primarily diagnosed in North America by DID experts who overdiagnose the disorder

3 DID is rare

4 DID is an iatrogenic disorder (suggested/caused by the treating clinician) rather than a trauma-based disorder

5 DID is the same entity as Borderline Personality Disorder

6 DID treatment is harmful to patients

After presenting the data to prove these claims as false, Brand and her colleagues assert that DID is present in about 1 percent of the general population, and DID actually remains under-recognized and undertreated. They state, "DID is a legitimate and distinct psychiatric disorder that is recognizable worldwide and can be reliably identified in multiple settings by appropriately trained researchers and clinicians." If you are in any situation, institutionally or within your own care as a client, where the legitimacy of how you present in the world is being negated, please get a copy of the Brand article online and present it to whoever might be challenging you. The data and the peer-reviewed studies do exist. And even though this more empirical work is not the focus of this book, we recognize that it may be important for you in engaging the advocacy that you need to do.

There are two other significant areas of controversy that come up in discussions around dissociation that I would also like to address in this section. The first myth involves the nature of trauma that must be present to develop a dissociative disorder in the first place. In graduate school, on the one day that DID was mentioned, the professor taught that only extended sexual trauma in a monstrous context like ritual Satanic abuse can possibly cause something like DID. Engaging in detailed discussions about the nature of ritual abuse and mind control extends beyond the scope of this book, suffice it to say that they are real and can be the reason that people present for help. Sandra Johnson, one of our contributors, disclosed her own experience with abuse of this nature in chapter 2. Susan Pease Banitt, who did hotline work for many years and fielded constant reports of this horrendous form of abuse, also attests to its reality and has actively fought against it for years, often at risk to her own professional reputation.

If you survived trauma of this nature, in seeking out a therapist it does become important to vet whom you will see and ask if they validate these forms of abuse and control as true. And if they seem trauma-competent but do not have specific training in working with ritual Satanic abuse, institutional mind control, or cultic abuse, ask if they are willing to receive consultation on the matter in working with your case. We provide further resources in this area in the Recommended Reading and Resources section. *However, we need to emphasize that the presence of DID or a dissociative disorder does not automatically mean that you or any other person experienced these kinds of abuses. All types of unhealed trauma can lead to dissociative disorders.* Although pervasive developmental trauma early in life is often seen with a DID diagnosis, even the character of that can differ from person to person (or system to system). So it's important that a therapist or any helper you see not make assumptions.

Another great myth that exists, which might better be described as a bias, is the notion that people with dissociative disorders (especially DID) are treatment-resistant and cannot live full lives. Although more on this matter is addressed in our Appendix for clinicians and therapists, we feel it's important to address it here in the general content as well because you may run into a therapist or helping professional in your pursuit of healing that's been impacted by this bias. Rachael, one of our contributors with dissociative features as part of complex trauma, said that her EMDR Therapy professional training literally "scared the shit" out of her around working with dissociation. She recalls, "If a person is dissociative do not touch them with a ten-foot pole, that's the message I got, and that needs to stop." In discussing these types of fears with our contributors, there is overwhelming consensus that they originate in mental health professionals' own fear of trauma and dissociation, generally stemming from not doing their own work or coming to terms with how trauma and dissociation play out in their lives. The *us versus them* divide and fears around not wanting to do more harm to clients if one does not know how to "bring them back" or "bring them out" of a dissociative experience can also play a role.

As I explained in the previous chapter's commentary on EMDR Therapy, I do believe that some screening and caution is prudent, especially for new or emerging therapists. Yet too often this caution gets communicated as, "This person cannot be helped because they are too dissociative." When screening for dissociative expressions is working at its best, a clinician will identify the level of dissociation they are dealing with in order to develop a plan. This plan ought to involve receiving consultation or extra help in training on a case while they learn more about the true nature of dissociation and not just operate on old myths or outdated information they might have received along the way. The best consultation will challenge willing professionals to look at their own biases and struggles and often inspire professionals to engage in more of their own trauma-focused work.

I wish I could say that this kind of attitude that Rachael encountered is the exception rather than the rule among therapists and clinicians. Yet I'm still hearing it in EMDR Therapy circles, just as frequently as when I myself was trained in 2005. I wish that clinical professionals, on the whole, were not skittish about treating dissociative disorders. I wish that the field and society at large could recognize that people with dissociative disorders, including those people with DID, are high functioning overall—because their dissociative gifts and their systems allow them to be. And I also wish there were more glimmers of hope out there. Yet Andrea, another one of our blended personal/professional contributors was still taught in her graduate program (2016–2017), more than a decade after mine, that DID and dissociative disorders are rare. There is still a problem with how dissociative disorders are perceived, not just by society, but by the field of the helping professions. And it's time we spoke truth about what's really going on.

What are all of these disputes really about? Although dissociation can show up in a wide range of clinical diagnoses, it's been clearly established that unhealed trauma is a major causal factor in the development of clinically significant dissociative disorders.[2] And drawing so much attention to the impact of trauma can make powerful people uncomfortable. This truth has been evident since the days of Freud (see chapter 1), and things might be looking even bleaker in modern times because current power structures rely on the dissociated nature of colonial patriarchy to function. And in these systems, holding the powerful accountable for traumatic injury is simply not acceptable.

If you are interested in learning more about this history and debate around dissociation, trauma, and memory, please read Anna Holtzman's excellent overview of the "memory wars" in the field of psychology. Full information about her article, "Harvey Weinstein's 'False Memory' Defense and Its Shocking Origin Story," appears in the Recommended Reading and Resources section. The memory wars refer to decades of debate in the field about the trustworthiness of memory, particularly as it relates to accusations of abuse by survivors of trauma. The subtitle of Holtzman's investigation conveys the essence of the problem: how powerful sex offenders manipulated the field of psychology. She discusses the history of the False Memory Syndrome Foundation, founded by the parents of Dr. Jennifer Freyd (a former president of the International Society for the Study of Trauma and Dissociation). Dr. Freyd accused her parents of abuse, and their response was to attempt to discredit survivors of abuse by unleashing this organization. Their organization sadly received the support of leaders in the field like Dr. Aaron Beck, a founder of CBT, and Dr. Elizabeth Loftus, the notorious "false memory" researcher who often appears as an expert witness for alleged perpetrators in court.[3]

Trauma and dissociation advocates declare that the memory wars are over and have been won, as the evidence presented in Holtzman's article supports. As long as unhealed trauma continues to plague society and people are threatened by its impact or made to feel responsible for it, there is a likelihood that such debate, even in scholarly settings, will continue. There are two international organizations for studying the impact of trauma that have remarkably similar names: The International Society for Traumatic Stress Studies (ISTSS) and the later-founded International Society for the Study of Trauma and Dissociation (ISSTD). Even the existence of two organizations of this nature paints a disturbing picture because many trauma advocates widely dismiss the existence of, or at least the full impact of, dissociation. And recall my experience with the EMDR Therapy community and what Rachael heard at her training on dissociation. Bear in mind these are EMDR trainers saying this, and EMDR is supposed to be one of the leading trauma-focused modalities available! While the answer of the ISSTD and mainstream advocates in the field of dissociation conduct research and scholarship to prove that dissociative disorders are real and treatable, there is still a concern by advocates like myself that such a focus may measure the experiences of survivors without adequately including our voices in the advocacy.

And that is where this book seeks to change the conversation.

Media Portrayal of Dissociation and Dissociative Disorders

Two competing narratives exist in society, both of which negate the essence of who people with dissociative disorders really are. The first, as we established, are largely academic presences who continually attempt to discredit the very real existence of dissociation and dissociative disorders. The other narrative, largely promoted by media, is that dissociative disorders do exist and that they are always the stuff of high drama and intrigue.

In late 2020, *The Mighty* published an article that I wrote aimed at the popular American director Ryan Murphy, asking him to consider how his portrayal of DID in his new series *Ratched* is damaging.[4] Ryan Murphy is one of my favorite creatives working today, and as a big fan of his work, I was hoping he could do something interesting, yet responsible, with his new series that told the backstory of Nurse Ratched of *One Flew Over the Cuckoo's Nest* fame. Yet when the character with DID at the mental hospital was introduced, of course she was the murderer. And of course they factored in her multiplicity, which was caused by abuse, as the source of her murderous rampages. This series aired in 2020. I am fed up, and so is my larger community of people with dissociative disorders, with how we are portrayed in movies and other media.

In 2022, during the final stages of my writing this book, Marvel (the cinematic universe for which I professed my love in chapter 4), took on DID portrayal in their new series *Moon Knight*. This TV series looked to a minor character in the Marvel canon whose superhero name is Moon Knight. His multiplicity was not just metaphorical or part of the alter ego device that appears throughout many fictional worlds. Rather, Mark/Steven, the protagonist, formed into a multiple system as a result of multilayered childhood loss and parental abuse. And a powerful god-figure took advantage of his woundedness and his fractured mind in order to get him to do that god's bidding.

And . . . you guessed it! That bidding included killing others.

Before I go on with my commentary, I must first acknowledge that several survivors of mind control programs—whether they were government-sponsored as in the case of the Central Intelligence Agency (CIA)'s MK-Ultra* from 1953–1973, or connected to various forms of ritual abuse—*may* have experiences closer to what is portrayed in the movies. I've both met and heard sharing over the years from people recruited into violence because of their woundedness, yet please bear in mind that this phenomenon can even play out with how mainstream military recruiters operate, which our contributor Jackson discussed in his interview. While I wholeheartedly validate that the experiences of those who have survived mind control may include being asked to harm others, I must also heartily assert that these experiences are not typical of people I've met or treated with dissociative disorders. And we must break the association at the societal level that dissociation automatically equals violence.

My heart broke watching *Moon Knight* because there was so much that Marvel got right. So many of Mark/Steven's experiences were incredibly real to me, as brilliantly acted by Oscar Isaac. They showed the development of a system and how an internal world can be experienced better than any attempt I've ever seen in the movies or on TV. I later discovered that Isaac read Robert Oxnam's well-known memoir *A Fractured Mind* to prepare.[5] There is even a scene of dialogue where Mark acknowledges that Steven, the alter/part formed to manage the abuse, is the real superpower! My emotional responses to watching so much of *Moon Knight* were very real, and yet whenever the assassin trope kept coming out, my heart deflated with that same old familiar sense of *here we go again*. . . . And this leads to the question: are these steps in

---

* To read and listen more about MK-Ultra, please go to this episode of NPR's *Fresh Air* with Terry Gross from September 9, 2019: www.npr.org/2019/09/09/758989641/the-cias -secret-quest-for-mind-control-torture-lsd-and-a-poisoner-in-chief.

the right direction still doing more harm than good, especially when so much misunderstanding about dissociation and multiplicity abounds?

As I discovered in preparing for this book, it's not just those of us with dissociative disorders who are frustrated. Ron Davis, a documentary filmmaker, found himself watching a documentary on the Discovery Channel about DID and felt there was more to the story that was not being captured. He knew that it was badly done and that there seemed to be no reason for the documentary other than sensationalism. He also recalled earlier features about DID on daytime talk shows like *Geraldo, Phil Donahue,* or *Sally Jessy Raphael* that were incredibly formulaic. These episodes would feature an abused woman who showed several different personalities (e.g., the big spender, the kid, the teenager). Ron recalls, "And then after break some wing nut therapist would come on trying to explain it all." Ron wanted to meet more people with dissociative disorders and shed light on the nuance of these stories, which is how he connected with the organization An Infinite Mind.

In developing his documentary project *I Am We,* which he worked on for six years, he deliberately wanted to choose someone to feature who would feel like "the neighbor next door" and not someone you would see on *Sally Jessy Raphael* or another daytime talk show. In describing Willow, the protagonist of his documentary, he said, "You wouldn't know on the surface that she has DID." For him, this *relatability* is paramount and is how we are going to change the conversation and get more widespread understanding of DID out there that is not sensationalized. Says Ron, "Sensationalism is entertaining and reality is less entertaining unless you find the right conduit for it." He believes that Willow, a middle-aged mother with a husband, two adult children, and a group of friends from the suburbs is the right conduit if you're going to break down stereotypes.

I saw *I Am We,* and my company even made a contribution toward its production. I believe it is another step in the right direction for how dissociative disorders are portrayed. I anticipate that there will inevitably be criticism from those of us seeking an even more normalized portrayal of DID in media because in the film there is so much switching shown, especially of Willow's littles. Personally, I thought it was well-done and respectful, and my Four connected very strongly and emotionally with one of Willow's very young parts.

Where I found myself wincing a little is when, in interviewing Ron, I heard him explain his process for finding a protagonist that is relatable. As the media voice in our collection of contributors, I truly wanted to listen to what he had to say. Yet it made me a bit angry that society at large would likely find a white, heteronormative woman who could be the "person next door" as the relatable candidate. Ron knows this as someone in the field of media and offered the insight very candidly for the interview. For me, even though I can appreciate *I Am We*, it shows me how much work still needs to be done, not just destigmatizing dissociation and mental illness. Rather, there is much work that needs to be done amplifying marginalized voices in our popular discourse and encouraging the mainstream to regard these voices just as valuably as we might that of a white woman from the suburbs. This might be easier said than done in a society that revolves around the dissociative nature of *us versus them* to function.

Social media has given people with dissociative disorders from a variety of backgrounds a platform to share their stories and to self-advocate. Many of the contributors I spoke with for the project, especially those who are part of online support groups for people with DID, are active consumers of this media. Dr. Emily Christensen (aka Emma Sunshaw) made a splash when her popular podcast *System Speak* debuted in 2017. Emily features a blend of expert guests (I had the privilege to appear in 2021) and sharing her own lived experience as a therapist managing her own DID. *System Speak* is one of the most widely recommended resources that we share with our clinical students and often our clients who want to learn more about dissociative disorders through a personal lens.

Although he is not the only one advocating in the larger sphere of social media, an individual with DID whose host, or primary adult part, is named Chris, has over a million followers on the popular app TikTok (@theasystem). The entire DID community on TikTok and YouTube was featured in a piece in *Input* magazine in 2021.[6] The piece raised some interesting questions about whether these social media communities are helpful for people with DID seeking support, or whether they've created a sea of *influencers* who are exploiting themselves or maybe even acting. While claims about people "faking" their DID are certainly not new, even I am aware that we're in an entirely new arena with the commercialese of modern social media—which is perhaps why I've never found it useful to check out many of these influencers. Yet if my clients find them useful, I would certainly be willing to use the content they connect with as a springboard for conversation. Interestingly, the article itself in *Input* was still filled with many of the same tropes that I've called out in this chapter; even though it correctly cited the adult prevalence of DID as being between 1–1.5 percent of the general population, they continued to call the condition "rare" or "a rarity."

European Journal of Trauma & Dissociation, a peer-reviewed journal, published a 2022 piece from *System Speak* creator Dr. Emily Christensen about the rise of online communities for people with DID and other dissociative expressions.[7] While Emily explores many facets of the issue in her article, she most importantly takes on the issue of whether such forums may be helpful or harmful to clients. She encourages people who are drawn to these groups, and therapists who are guiding them, to examine whether the content of these groups and social media platforms are focused on healing and recovery (which is optimal) or whether they seem focused on sharing horror stories and retellings of trauma narratives. While the latter may play some role in validating people's experiences, extended exposure to such content can be chronically triggering and ultimately unhelpful without some type of healing solution promoted. One of my associates who works with adolescents made the comment that TikTok seems to be a reason why so many teenagers now think that they have DID. While such media can lead to productive conversations between young clients and their therapists about the normal nature of parts and what constitutes parts constellations leading to problems of living or even diagnoses, time will tell whether the social media element has done more harm than good for advocacy.

Occasionally there is good attention paid by media when a celebrity mentions their connection to DID—although there have not been many such instances. AnnaLynne McCord, whose quote opens the chapter, is an actress who came out in early 2021 with her own DID diagnosis. Supported in interviews by her consulting physician Dr. Daniel Amen, McCord revealed that her younger part or alter revealed itself when she was preparing for a role. Whatever you might think of her or how she is advocating, when she said she is *absolutely uninterested in shame* upon revealing her diagnosis, I was impressed. My system rejoiced for her.

There have only been a few other substantive disclosures of celebrities with DID, including comedian Roseanne Barr and former NFL player Herschel Walker, who penned his own memoir *Breaking Free: My Life with Dissociative Identity Disorder* in 2009. Perhaps I am biased because I do not support their political beliefs and publicity stunts, but I have not observed much substantial evidence that their coming out has forwarded the conversation or changed the narrative. Other celebrities have referenced having "multiple personality disorders" or alter egos, although many of these comments seem to come across as more joking in nature. There are online accounts that surmise that many high-drama celebrities, both those who are alive and those who are deceased, may have/had a DID diagnosis.

Of the celebrity accounts around dissociative disorders, I've most closely and interestedly followed the disclosures of Adam Duritz, lead singer of the band Counting Crows. Duritz first came out in 2008 with his diagnosis of Depersonalization, which he describes as a condition that "makes you look at life from a distance," although he maintains it's affected him his entire life.[8] Some of the interviews and insights he's given online through the years, which can be obtained via a simple search, are beautifully candid and profound. I encourage you to check them out, especially if you connect with his music. Full disclosure: Jamie fell in love with Counting Crows when we were chronologically nineteen (1998–1999), and perhaps our Nineteen part remains connected to their music because it was there for her at a time when she needed someone to see her the most. We get chills whenever we think about this dissociatively creative connection to Adam Duritz and how it pieced together so many years later. . . .

Our Contributors Speak

A general consensus among our contributors is that the way media handles the portrayal of dissociation needs to change. Heather (LS) Scarboro+ asserts, "There should be a law prohibiting any misinformation that is put out there about mental illnesses, especially DID." There is also some recognition that if one high-profile person came out about their dissociative disorder, it might create some kind of shift. Yet several contributors recognize the problem with celebrity culture and acknowledge that change must start with our own willingness to come out, to be public, and to have these difficult conversations. And in these conversations we must assert that using terms like *split personality* or *multiple personalities* is no longer helpful. Rather, we must encourage people at large to recognize that dissociation applies to all of us in one way or another. This sense of normalization may help to promote greater understanding of how and why people may struggle. Destiny Aspen Mowadeng would like to see more widespread acceptance of a *social model of disability* instead of a medical one.* In Destiny's words, "The world external to us and its barriers are what create our disabilities not our physical bodies; versus the medical model that

---

* Destiny highly recommends this YouTube video from advocate Molly Burke that explains the differences between the social and medical models of disability: https://youtu.be/aPEuYrtuxEk. She also recommends this video for how it applies to DID from The Ring System: www.youtube.com/watch?v=5KHdY5GoJJ4

sees us as entirely one-dimensional diagnoses." Because barriers to adequate treatment and understanding come from external societal factors, encouraging people to recognize that dissociation applies to all of us in one way or another can normalize the idea and create better conditions overall.

The Garden System, in expressing their concern even about more responsible portrayals of DID in media, states that viewers can leave with a sense of "Oh that poor person," instead of seeing how dissociation can work wonders in their life. Many contributors believe that the conversation around dissociation at a public level needs to involve more about the strengths and gifts of having a dissociative mind and not just focus on the maladaptive elements. The concluding chapter that follows focuses exclusively on these gifts as shared by our contributors. Katarina Lundgren says, "Take the [final] *D* off of DID when we talk about it publicly. More emphasis on dissociative experiences." For Dr. Kellie Kirksey, "Dissociation keeps people sane and safe enough; more talk about this, please."

Dr. Kirsten Koenig adds, "Dissociation is not what people think—dissociation does not have to be bad, sometimes it can keep you alive. When people can understand it without a label, there is less judgment involved. But we tend to label every little thing. To allow people to have the freedom if they need to, and give them the help to come back to this body when they need to—make it a place that's safe to come back to."

Cheryl, our contributor who carries both a DID diagnosis and a schizoaffective disorder diagnosis, shared a very powerful reflection with me about the role of media after our interview. She wrote,

> The media's continued portrayal of people with DID as men who are serial killers who are faking DID does thousands of traumatized women, like myself, a huge disservice. DID is not what people think it is. It's not overt and dramatic switches or a get out of jail free card. The majority of DID sufferers are women who have been so severely traumatized that we don't even remember it consciously. Can't remember. DID is finding a used hair accessory (presumably off the ground) that I've never seen before on the floor of my locked car after a shop at Wal-Mart and feeling a rush of terror because I have no memory of it but it must have been me. It's needing a system of Post-its and alarms to make sure everything is remembered. DID is being terrified of my 6'5" tall boss, even though he's the absolute nicest guy. DID is setting my tea on the roof of my car and a second later waking from a 'nap' in the parking lot at my work. It's disorienting and confusing and extremely painful. It's having different ways of being that are all a part of myself and yet strangely separate and compartmentalized.

For Elizabeth Davis, it saddens her that so many professional clinicians have shame about their own dissociative disorders or dissociative tendencies being known. What makes it more of a shame, says Elizabeth, is that so many clinicians get into this field because of their own lived experiences with trauma. She sees book projects like this one as vital in creating space for clinicians to be human. And that is a critical factor in removing stigma. John Fugett feels that this shift will happen one day, but it will take time. Clinicians, and society at large, fundamentally need to move past a worldview where the cognitive takes supremacy, and really get into our emotional worlds from which we are so dissociated. John reflects, "Our emotional self goes to our actual experience if we'll listen to it."

John's commentary about the dissociation between our cognitive and emotional selves is the primary reason I see in why professionals can continue to discount the existence of dissociation. Or why well-intentioned professionals can be so afraid of treating it, or of coming out regarding their own struggles. In a world where fully experiencing emotion can still be seen as weak or terrifying, it can seem safer to retreat into the realm of the neocortex and never once connect with our emotions, our heart, and our body. Or perhaps we connect with them only in private and never feel safe enough to bring them out to play. I'm not saying that the cognitive realm is inherently evil—in many ways it is protective and can help us get things done in our lives. In my experience, that cognitive realm is largely what drives the Dr. Jamie part of my identity. Yet if she stayed in control too much or too long, the emotional wonder and zest for life that is Jamie would never get to come through.

Being Agents for Change in Dissociated Systems

Several contributors, like Dianne Harper, saw their engagement with this interview and this book project as a vital part of their coming-out process. We truly believe that if dissociative disorders are going to be taken more seriously while not being sensationalized, those of us with dissociative experiences of life must be willing to come out and advocate. More stories. More voices. More faces. More experiences from different kinds of people.

As I explained in the introduction, coming out was a process for me, and I was fearful at times because of the stigma around dissociation. I also feel it was important for me to come out in baby steps. With every level of privilege I attained in my career, the more responsibility I felt to speak up. Yet with that privilege comes a great deal of insulation from harm that I recognize not everyone has at every stage of their career. So how you disclose your dissociative disorder or any other mental health condition is fundamentally a personal choice where you must take many variables into account—above all, your own safety. One of our contributors added anonymously, "People are judgey. This is a reason I will not tell my family that I have DID, afraid that they're going to do their own Internet research."

Amy Wagner, my personal friend, professional collaborator, and bastion of wisdom about her dissociative experience of life, believes we need to normalize the human experience and all be able to look at our professional capacity. Yet she tells quite the horror story about how her eagerness to be transparent about her DID during both her graduate program and her first internship site seemed to backfire on her. Amy remembers, "That was a mistake. For the rest of my program I felt like I was held to a higher standard and was the topic of staff meetings. There were subtle, hurtful comments that came through on papers. It was the same at my internship site. There was no room for my humanity."

Olga Trujillo acknowledges that even though they are out about their journey with DID, some professions can be more brutal than others in allowing a person to be fully human. Being out as a judge, a lawyer, or someone in law enforcement might be next to impossible. It's hard enough for clinical professionals to be out about their struggles with DID. I can't even imagine how difficult it might be for people in professions that actively promote dissociation from emotion and humanity as part of their cultural norms. So assessing whether it is safe to come out in your professional life is a first step that many people navigate.

Olga explains that even though it is illegal for a person to be fired based solely on their diagnosis, institutions can find clever ways to "get rid of someone" if they really want them gone. This campaign typically involves scrutinizing elements like attendance and performance; as Amy noted, *being held to a higher standard.* Many clinical professionals I've spoken to over the years express fear over coming out in any public way, or even sharing their diagnosis with clients in the spirit of appropriate self-disclosure, fearing retribution or retaliation. The issue of disclosing to clients, if you are a clinical professional, is one that we discuss in general as helping professionals—whether or not dissociation is involved. The overall teaching I adhere to is that if there is some evident therapeutic value for sharing parts of your journey with your client, it can be warranted. Yet self-disclosing never ought to be about you working out your stuff with your client. If you are a client and your therapist shares quite a bit about their life, you have every right to tell them whether it is helpful to your process, or if you prefer that they not talk about themselves so much.

I've heard on more than one occasion from clinical professionals, which include a few of our contributors, that their biggest fear is being reported to their state licensing board as impaired. If one's license ends up being suspended or revoked, that can impact one's livelihood. And even if a license is never suspended or revoked, the investigation process can feel shaming and re-traumatizing. Because this fear is consistently articulated by my colleagues who want to come out—either to their clients or at a more public level—I decided to investigate for myself how things might be handled in my home state of Ohio if someone ever decided to report me as impaired.

At the time that one applies for their first clinical license in Ohio, they are required to disclose impairment or treatment for any clinical diagnoses. Typically as long as evidence of treatment is provided there is no issue, and this was the case for me in 2005. I must admit, when I published some of my more provocative articles over the years, including my coming-out piece in 2018 and a piece I wrote at the beginning of the COVID-19 pandemic admitting to still having fleeting episodes of suicidal ideation, I had some low-grade anxiety that someone might judge me as impaired and report me to my board. Even when I was going through my divorce, I feared that my ex-husband might add contacting the board to his list of retaliatory tactics. And yes, when I reached out to the chief ethics investigator and director of the State of Ohio Counselor, Social Worker, and Marriage and Family Therapist Board to inquire about their willingness to speak to me for the book, my heart fluttered with some nerves. Hitting "send" on the email caused my throat to drop a bit. Even as well-established Dr. Jamie Marich, I had a sense of, "You're giving them too much about yourself by sharing your diagnosis and work this openly. They might use it against you."

Our board director, deputy director, and chief ethics investigator met with me over Zoom as part of this book preparation process to discuss some of my concerns and those I shared on behalf of my colleagues. They assured me that they are used to screening out complaints from people like disgruntled ex-spouses or former colleagues that seem to be retaliatory in nature. Furthermore, the only real grounds that they have to move on a complaint is if evidence exists that a professional's mental health or recovery concerns (i.e., impairment) are impacting client care or well-being. They also assured me that there is due process with the investigation, and if it does get to the level where a licensee needs to be clinically evaluated for treatment, the licensee does have a say in who is conducting the evaluation. Typically these evaluations come at the expense of the licensee, which can add to the shame and frustration of the process, especially if a complaint is unfounded. I shared with my board representatives that when dissociative disorders and DID are involved, I wanted them to be aware that many clinical professionals, especially psychiatrists, still operate with outdated and biased information about DID. They seemed to hear me and assured me that a licensee with a dissociative disorder would not be randomly assigned to an evaluator without their consent and input.

If you in any way fear that your being more public about your diagnosis might have ramifications for your license (regardless of your profession) or your livelihood, I encourage you to do your homework and even to consult a lawyer. At the very least, consider discussing your desire to come out or be more vocal in some way with your own therapist so they can advocate for you if needed. Some of you might not feel like this is necessary, but if these barriers around your employment and how you are received are getting in the way, consider accessing this assistance. One of our contributors reports that her diagnosis has often been used against her, especially by Child Protective Services, in custody proceedings. So know your rights, which can also involve reaching out to disability advocacy organizations in your state. Here in my state, I have Disability Ohio on speed dial in case I ever need them.

The greatest fears about coming out may involve navigating your own shame and how you see yourself in relation to your diagnosis. If this idea resonates with you, seek out support from your personal therapist or helping professional to discuss the risks and benefits of coming out. Working through any layers that exist on the surface of that decision about honoring yourself and your journey can prove very valuable to your healing process. Seeking support from friends, online support groups for people with DID (including several tailored to professionals with DID), or from organizations like An Infinite Mind might also be options. An Infinite Mind does an excellent job of keeping their conference sites as private as possible, and going over guidelines to assure participant privacy and confidentiality. Jaime Pollack and her team are diligent in assuring these safeguards, fully aware that not everyone who comes to the annual conference is able to be out in all aspects of their lives.

These resources might also link you with other people who have come out in one or more areas of their lives—to their families, professionally, or on social media. I am happy to be the person who offers my lived experience to others about what coming out with a dissociative disorder has been like for me, and my personal therapist, Elizabeth Davis, has been with me every step of the way. In her interview for this project, I asked her if she had any concerns about me coming out with my diagnosis, or if any concerns have surfaced for her since. She honestly answered no, but then turned the question around on me to ask if anything has surprised me about coming out that feels concerning. My honest answer is that I was not expecting to be inundated with so many emails and messages from people reaching out and asking for help and guidance. Such messages continue to this day, and I expect they'll be even more numerous after this book is published.

On one hand, I am honored and consider it a privilege that putting myself out there has facilitated a trust where people, especially clinical professionals, can come to me and say *me too*. I will never forget the day when Katharine, one of our contributors whom I first met as a clinical student in a training course, came to me over break and told me that she had DID. She punctuated this disclosure with, "I've never told another professional that, ever. I thought I never would. You being so open about yours has helped me realize I have to do this."

Yet on the other hand, it can be draining having so much of one's self (or selves) out there like that. I believe in the power of radical vulnerability to engender change, but even with the boundaries I've put on my sharing, it's tough. I follow my first recovery sponsor's guidance of not sharing in the public forum what I haven't spent some time working through therapeutically first, and I try to keep the emphasis of my sharing more on the recovery and less on the trauma. Many people who message me feel they know me better than they really do, and others seem to rely on me too much because they feel I'm the first person who has truly understood them. The reality is I cannot be everyone's therapist and even with help answering messages (thanks to our contributor Alicia Hann), I/we can only do so much.

Does any of what I just shared make me regret coming out?

Absolutely not.

I will say I've learned a great deal more about the importance of taking care of myself and the deep necessity of rest. Boundaries are also a part of what we generally call self-care, or what I prefer to think of as self-nourishment. As an example, I no longer keep Facebook on my phone. I also make sure to schedule several days each month when I am not on the computer and am truly doing what I as *Jamie* wants to do. My evening time, when I can just take a walk without my phone or watch television is also essential to my well-being.

So if you are planning to come out in any substantial way or work as an advocate for the needs of others, please be mindful of exhausting yourself. We need you, but not at the expense of your own health.

Chuck Bernsohn—whose experiences with dissociation exist at the intersection of their chronic pain/disability, being trans, and living with ADD—believes that aside from big systemic changes, personal responsibility is also vital. Chuck says, "It's important to be as transparent as feels safe to me about my mental health." When I asked Chuck to expound upon what safety means for them, they said, "A moment in which I can share of myself without losing connection to another person or losing connection to that part of myself."

BeeJay recognizes that there are still a lot of systems who feel the need to hide, yet BeeJay also draws hope seeing more and more systems that are out there and speaking up.

Melissa Parker, another therapist with DID, believes that us coming out, speaking up, and telling our own stories is imperative to creating change, especially for clinical professionals. Says Melissa, "We need to burn the mental health system down and start over. But since we can't do that, we need more voices of lived experience in the field. We need to rewrite the language. It's hard to get rid of stigma while we [in the field] are using horrible language and the so-called experts are saying such things about us." Things like "screening out dissociation in evaluating treatment," comments like Dr. Frank Anderson's about people with Dissociative Identity Disorder being "masters of deception,"[9] and denials of dissociation's existence in some circles—these are merely a short list of what Melissa encapsulates in her comment.

The Native and Indigenous perspectives offered in this book would suggest that we have to build circles or bridges instead of defined walls; Julian Jaramillo and Wayne William Snellgrove both spoke to this idea in their interviews. Malika believes, "Educating people who have been through trauma is good, educating people who haven't been through it can be very supportive." Adam O'Brien, a cisgender white male, recognizes that in increasing our understanding of dissociation we must listen more fully to women, to Native people, to marginalized people—people, he says, "who are closer to the heart."

So how do we facilitate that connection when people on the other side of the bridge may have no desire to really get to know us?

We've contemplated this question throughout Dr. Jamie's professional career and wish we had something brilliant to offer you. Yet some days we find ourselves in tears wondering if building these bridges will ever be possible.

And we feel like we're letting you down by not ending the chapter with some grand conclusion. So here is an insight from Jamie's life that might give us something. . . .

In the summer of 2021, I sat in a chapel run by a major religious order before the Holy Mass, where my brother (whom I dearly love) would make his vows of Solemn Profession, his next step on his way to ordination as a Roman Catholic priest. A great, conflicting pain overcame me in those moments before the Mass, a pain that says, "You belong here, and you don't." The part of me that has always felt at home in a Catholic setting is that love of the ritual and ceremony, the smell of the incense, the familiarity of the chants and songs. When I sink into these, I feel connected to my Croatian ancestors and our Catholic faith. And even though I don't fully believe every word of the Nicene Creed as it relates to Jesus, I certainly feel connection to Christ Consciousness. I've always been cool with Jesus—it's his followers that can piss me off. And therein exists the other part of the conflict—I am queer, bisexual, and an advocate for other queer and transgender people to live the fullest, most open expressions of themselves in all spaces of life, especially faith-based spaces. As a survivor, I can't sit in a Catholic Church and not feel uneasy about the legacy of abuse and silencing survivors within the Church. Between my queer identity and dedication to supporting survivors no matter what, I truly feel that I don't belong.

So in those moments before the Mass, with all these deep feelings swirling me into a frenzy, I made a bold decision: I decided to sing with all my heart. Literally sing. It would be the only way that I could keep from destructively dissociating and potentially imploding during the Mass. The nice thing about Mass in traditional settings is the brilliant *schola* (Latin chant choir) and in this case it was populated by my brother's fellow priests and brothers. Adding my voice to theirs somehow felt like my way of saying, "I am a woman, and my voice belongs here too."

I chanted the Mass setting, *Missa Cum Jubilo,* not missing a beat of the Latin. Having been a liturgical music director as one of my many jobs back when I worked in Medjugorje, Bosnia-Herzegovina during my service there from 2000–2003, I got quite good at reading and singing it. And I love it. Comfort comes to me through these sacred tones.

I actually felt very good after the Mass, being able to fully engage in the celebratory dinner for my brother because I had just spent close to an hour singing. But then later in the day one of my brother's very traditional, conservative friends who sat near me during the Mass said, "Wow, you really sing Latin beautifully. I didn't think that was something *you* would know how to do."

Her tone said it all, and my stomach dropped a bit.

Maintaining my calm, I responded, "Well, I do have a background in liturgy, and singing has always been my favorite part of the Mass."

She politely nodded, not really knowing what to say to that.

What I really wanted to say is, "Yes, queer, liberal, feminist, 'nonreligious' people can love Jesus too. We can sing. We can talk theology. And maybe even with more gusto than you because we've actually used sacred ritual to embrace our human experience, not try to push it away."

Yet I've learned that saying such things to people who don't want to hear them usually only works me up even more. So I just sing anyway. . . .

I feel similarly now as I wrap up this chapter leading toward the conclusion of this book—a book that is truly a love letter to my own dissociative mind and hopefully a vehicle for giving others like me a platform. As my first client with DID told me, "People fear what they don't understand," and over the years I've come to edit that slightly as, "People fear what they *won't* understand." There are people who will not care, there are people who will never meet us on the bridge halfway. And I'm not going to injure myself by always crossing the bridge to meet them and shake them into awareness, only to come back further depleted.

So I sing. I share. I offer my story and my experience, strength, and hope.

The people who are drawn to the song will hear it and perhaps be motivated to make some changes or sing out with their own stories too.

And just imagine what could happen if so many more of us sang anyway. . . .

Perhaps the sheer vibratory power of such a chorus would indeed change the world.

═══ EXPRESSIVE ARTS PRACTICE: WRITING A PITCH ═══

Exploring the problems with how media portrays dissociative disorders was a major theme in this chapter. In this expressive arts practice, you are invited to literally propose a new narrative. Imagine you are writing a pitch for a new movie, television series, or documentary to the head of a network. You have complete creative control to design this movie, series, or documentary however you want. If pitching a topic directly related to dissociation or dissociative disorders doesn't feel relevant to you, please considering using another mental health or recovery issue as the focus of your pitch.

Here are some areas that we suggest you include in your pitch:

- Tell us about the main characters, the supporting characters, or in the case of a documentary, any protagonists or issues of focus.

- What might be some of the main plot points or focus points you intend to explore in your work?

- What are some key reasons you believe the network ought to pick up this movie, series, or documentary?

- Who is the ideal demographic for watching your movie, series, or documentary? What audience are you writing this for?

In the spirit of expressive arts, if you'd like to design a cover poster for the series you are pitching, go ahead and create that. Let it show some of the themes you intend to explore in your creative work that will help you tell a new story in media.

⸺QUESTIONS TO ASK MY THERAPIST OR PSYCHIATRIST⸺

- What are your feelings about the way dissociative disorders, especially DID, are portrayed in the media?

- Have you ever considered anything you see in the movies or television to be a legitimate part of your training?

- What books or memoirs have you read by people with dissociative disorders or other mental health issues?

- What do you see as the number one reason there remains such stigma around mental health issues, especially those connected to trauma and dissociation?

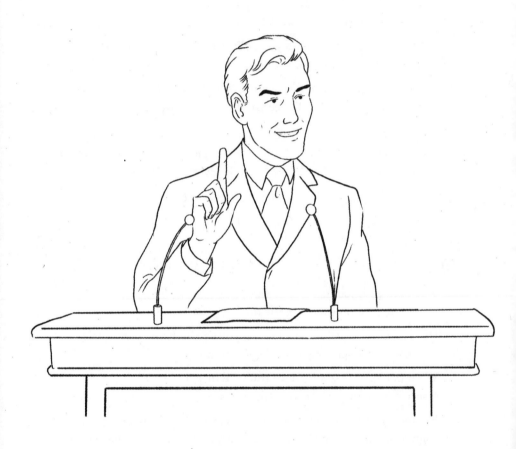

Conclusion

The Gifts of Dissociation

The things that make us different—those
are our superpowers.
—LENA WAITHE

Without any prompting from me, fifteen of our contributors used the word
superpower to describe their dissociative tendencies and gifts. While we generally view superpowers as the stuff of fantasy, mythology, or even the paranormal, they are so much more than that. Lena Waithe, a performer and the
first African American woman to win an Emmy award for comedy writing,
frames it well in this chapter's opening quote. Our superpowers are anything
that make us different, and a hopeful theme that's come through in this book
is that *different is good.* Not only that, different is amazing! Different has helped
us to survive—and now for many of us, our differences and unique sensibilities allow us to thrive in our lives.

I am sure that many of you might be puzzled by the title of this chapter. If you're new to approaching your trauma and its evolving dissociative expressions, you might have a difficult time identifying anything as being positive right now, let alone being a gift. I think all of our contributors were there at one point or another, so we certainly honor that. We also hope that you can read on and listen to what some of our contributors have to say about how they've learned to make dissociation work for them in their lives, and how navigating their trauma recovery has allowed them to see their world in new ways.

One of our contributors who dissociates but does not have DID made the comment that DID has obviously protected many people from unspeakable horrors. Yet overall this contributor feels that the lives of people with DID would be better and easier without so much fragmentation to manage. I have to admit, I got a little defensive when I heard this comment, yet I want to acknowledge it as a feeling you might have at this point in the book. Even if you struggle with the impact of unhealed trauma and dissociation, it can be difficult to see the gifts, especially in a society that continues to pathologize emotional expression and stigmatize seeking help for mental health. So in this concluding chapter, which is also a response to comments shared by several contributors in chapter 7 calling for less focus on the *disorder* part of DID or dissociation, let's go there. Let's explore what our contributors have to say about the gifts of dissociation, and then we'll take this dance into a final call to action for all of our readers.

From the Lived Experience of Our Superheroes

When contributor Amy Wagner spoke to me about the unconditional support of her adult daughter Samantha, I immediately wanted to speak to Samantha about the experience of being raised by someone with DID. Samantha, who told me many times throughout the interview that she simply has an "amazing mom," believes it is ridiculous to assume that people with DID cannot be good parents. Of Amy's parenting, Samantha says, "She's so loving, so affectionate. When we were little, she was always wanting to play with us and has always been down to do whatever interests my brother and me in our lives." Samantha says that Amy did not give her a big "reveal" about having DID, it was more of an evolving conversation that happened over the years and is still happening. She did notice that when Amy started getting more significant mental health help, that the material—or connections to her past—were coming up quicker for her. Yet Samantha, who was in her teens at that time, embraced an attitude of willingness to learn.

Samantha is a professional golfer who hopes one day to play in the LPGA. She also offered us some interesting perspective on dissociation and how athletes use it to their benefit. She says, "It's common in the sports world, it's just not talked about. There are more people than not using dissociation, and I use it to thrive on the golf course." Samantha, who works with a swing coach who used to teach Annika Sörenstam of Sweden, mentioned Annika as an athlete who publicly speaks about dissociation. Curious, I set out on a search and was indeed amazed just how much Sörenstam, regarded as one of the greatest female golfers of all time, has spoken about dissociation in the press.

In a 2020 piece from *The Guardian* focusing on athlete mental health, Sörenstam joked that she never hit a bad shot in her life because she doesn't remember them! She relayed, "You've got to learn how to dissociate—make a quick analysis, boom. Forget about it, move on, don't carry it with you, learn from your mistakes. We all hit bad shots. It's just—how do you regain composure?"[1]

For many of our contributors, their ability to dissociate and know how to make use of its potential can help them do what Sörenstam speaks to; but not just on a golf course, also in the arena that is life. And you may be surprised to learn that for the people we spoke with for this project, it can be the dissociative gifts, not just the grounding or anchoring, that keep them composed in stressful or triggering situations. Let's hear what they have to say....

Adaptive Qualities of Dissociation

Every contributor noted something about their dissociative mind that they see, at the very least, as adaptive. The most common report is that their mind helps them accomplish a great deal in life. In Amy Wagner's words, "I get shit done like it's nobody's business because of my group that lives inside of me." She goes on to say, "The length of my life will not be enough to experience all of my gifts of dissociation; there is so much richness and curiosity. Time is linear and dissociation is not." Katharine's comments about the utility of her system reverberate with Amy's insights. Says Katharine, "If one of my parts doesn't understand something, another part does. This definitely makes me more empathetic as a counselor." Cheryl identifies as a very good problem solver because one of her more authoritarian parts can be counted on to say "is it useful?" to her when she is weighing possible solutions. Amy Brickler adds, "The positive of dissociation is that those intense emotions that probably would have killed me were siphoned out or taken by my system. But if I had to deal with all of those emotions myself all at one time, I think I'd permanently be at the state mental hospital as a resident. And I don't believe I could function with all that burden on me."

Paula S. contends that having dissociative gifts allows you to keep functioning in your daily life, even when it seems that the world is crashing in around you. She explains that it's helpful for her that she can put grief and stress aside temporarily when it's not the time to deal with it. She says, "I like that I can intentionally choose when I go in to process my feelings." Rebecca agrees, commenting that dissociation can allow her to be "in a zone," which is helpful when she's going through something terrible. She can come through as unscathed as possible and not have so much "cleanup" work to do on the other side. For Christy Dunn, "It's the glue that's allowed me to continue to survive and not completely fall apart, especially as a highly sensitive person." Alicia Hann agrees that dissociation helps her function in society. She also thinks of her system as protective, and being able to talk about her parts helps her go deeper into trauma work. For Kylie, who identifies as highly sensitive and easily overwhelmed, dissociation helps her not be as overwhelmed, which means she can leave things behind when she needs to. This skill is important for therapists who might become easily activated or absorbed into what their clients share, and it helps many of us therapists hold the best boundaries possible for our own care.

John Fugett describes dissociation as something that allows him to be in almost any scenario and look like he was born into it. Dissociation allows him to blend in, which he does admit has its downsides. The downside is that it feels like you are lacking a sense of self; the upside is that it can allow you to be present for potentially stressful activities like moving and traveling.

For Jackson, dissociation permits a "psychological distancing from all of the struggle and the pain, the corrosions from having to live in the corrosions of society." He further notes that his love of reggae music allows him to engage in this task, and it's no wonder to him that navigating the stressors of the COVID-19 pandemic led him to reconnect with reggae. In navigating chronic illness Chuck Bernsohn says that dissociation can be an effective tool for dealing with boredom, although they sometimes need to discern where the line exists between dissociation and avoidance. Destiny Aspen Mowadeng adds, "Dissociation gives me a felt sense of safety in a lot of ways if I disconnect."

Heather (LS) Scarboro+ simply says, "The creativity! It's always going. There is a sense of freedom within me." This creativity, or what one of our anonymous contributors calls his inner landscape he escaped to that is populated with imaginary worlds, can engender survival. Our contributor notes, "I had to dissociate in this way to survive." Andrea echoes, "I'm good at surviving and getting my needs met." On the topic of creativity, Sarah Smith notes, "I can use creativity differently. It keeps me from having to push everything and everyone away." Another anonymous contributor explains that creativity helps her be an excellent problem solver, which shows up well for her in both her professional and personal life.

The majority of contributors, like John and Chuck above, did note that there is often a fine line to negotiate between a dissociative response being adaptive and maladaptive. Malika contends that when dissociation is unconscious or just happens she can feel disempowered, but feels very empowered when she can actively choose to use it for her advantage. Blaise Harris adds, "Of course this shell can protect me from getting into trouble, which is critical as a Black man living in this society. Yet sometimes what I do to dissociate, like constantly going into helper mode with people or constantly being busy, the less I thought about the shit I needed to work on." Blaise also reflects, in considering his healing process that's helped him to identify these patterns, "It's okay if you're damn struggling. You don't have to do this shit by yourself. There are people who are willing, able, and capable to help you work through what you need to go through." Elizabeth Davis, one of the contributors who shared about her personal journey yet who also specializes in the treatment of dissociation and has guided countless people with dissociative issues through EMDR Therapy, notes that dissociative minds can see and find details in the world. She says, "Survivor-focused talents can be turned into skills. So how can we bring balance and treat the toxicity but allow the skills to remain?"

What Dissociation Can Allow for in Life

In Holli Ellis's experience, disconnection can lead to connection. She says that having spent so much time of her life in disconnection, she takes nothing for granted now and aims to create connections that bring her a sense of peace. Erin says, "If you can differentiate between a trauma response and intuition, the whole world is at your fingertips." Both Holli and Erin offer some insight into Elizabeth's question in the previous section—how can we treat the toxicity but allow the skills to remain? Both Holli and Erin reported healing work in many modalities that now allows them to differentiate, and ultimately put things into a greater sense of perspective for them and their systems. The process of how to arrive at this place is different for everyone.

Fiona exclaims, "I am continually amazed by how I can do things that make no sense, and I shouldn't be able to do it. I shouldn't be a therapist, I shouldn't be as well-adjusted as I am!" Jaime Pollack believes that her dissociative mind led her to be the successful person she is. It allowed her to be successful in high school and college, and helped her build her career and professional success. For Megan, dissociation allows her to see things from multiple sides and different perspectives. As an example, certain parts can do the speaking and teaching well for her. Julian Jaramillo believes that the good parts of dissociation helped him accommodate to living in the United States after emigrating from Ecuador. To Jacqueline Lucas, dissociation has a negative connotation but it can be very helpful for some people. It allows her to escape certain levels of physical pain and gives her the capacity to take a time-out, especially when she is overstimulated.

Danielle is very candid about what dissociation allowed her to do during a stressful 2020–2021, a time when she says that "life on life's terms was relentless." She goes on, "I didn't relapse or end up in a psychiatric hospital because of my ability to sever and compartmentalize as needed to continue to show up for myself and for my family."

For Rachael, a contributor who shared personally and is also a therapist, "Dissociation allows me to move through the world still seeing the best in people, to look for the good. The small parts before they were wounded allow me to see that." Rachael says that when she began her career as a therapist, she had doubts about whether she'd be able to work with people effectively, and now she

"Dissociation filled the shoes of a lot of things I was missing."

—PAULA

"Most people think it's bad but it can save your life."   —CRYSTAL

"You can still have a very fulfilling, successful life with DID."

—THE GARDEN SYSTEM

"If you are out there and you have DID, you're gonna make it, keep working on it. If the counselor you have isn't a fit for you, go and look for someone else. You do what you need to do for yourself even if your family or religious organization discourages it. You know in your gut what you need."   —KATHLEEN knows that she can. A.J. adds that she has a "way higher tolerance for weirdness" compared to her other friends, noting that people with dissociative disorders are comfortable with high levels of empathy because of the disparate perspectives in their own minds. Dianne Harper believes that being dissociative has made her much more compassionate and aware. Even from what she describes as a relative place of privilege as a white woman, she has some sense of awareness about the struggle and how hard it can be for people to "be" in the world.

Dianne says, "I have a core of steel. I can do anything. I can handle pretty much anything because I already have." Sandra adds, "Dissociation is an altered state that a lot of people have to take chemicals to get to and I do not." For Dr. Kirsten Koenig, the interplay can still cause an internal fight. She offers, "I've struggled with being here even though I've chosen to truly experience humanity in this lifetime." TaNiya speaks to the need to start trusting her dissociative gifts, saying, "Now that I'm starting to trust them, they are absolutely a super power."

What Our Contributors Would Like You to Know

For many of our contributors, getting interviewed for this book felt like they were being given a platform. To conclude this section, we decided to feature several of our contributors telling you—both members of the general public reading this book out of interest and those of you feeling a connection to the material—what they would most like you to know about themselves and their lives as people with dissociative minds.

"Dissociation has allowed me to not take myself so seriously and help others to recognize it in themselves. Dissociation helped me to survive the traumas and the emotions that I used to see as scary, and now I am able to help my clients recognize it in themselves because I have been there, I've experienced it, I know healing is a process and IS possible."

—MICHELLE KAHL

"Story and dissociation have been pathologized. Let's redefine therapy, have conversations, be out loud!"　　　　　—DR. KELLIE KIRKSEY

"I'm not hurt by dissociation, I'm hurt by other people and how they talk to me when I am dissociating."

—KATARINA LUNDGREN

A Final Call to Action for All Readers

Although he was not a formal contributor for the book, I frequently checked in with my former student, now friend and team member in my EMDR Therapy training program, Sam Ore. Sam is a white therapist from Montana who works on the Confederated Salish and Kootenai tribal reservation near Polson. Like many Montana therapists I know, including contributor Brandon Spangler, Sam is open-minded and open-hearted in learning from Native people. In my estimation, this cultural humility makes therapists like Sam and Brandon more attuned and trauma-informed with all the people they serve. And Sam has been thinking a great deal more about dissociation in this past year.

He observes, "It's incredible that our whole culture doesn't have a basic understanding of dissociation. I feel that if I had some basic understanding when I was in middle school, I probably could have prevented a lot of maladaptive patterns. I think that the idea of educating around mindfulness is great, yet much of the education that I received around mindfulness left out tracking my own dissociative patterns."

It sounds like Sam is suggesting that we all learn how to do Dissociative Profile exercises, and from as young of an age as possible!

I certainly feel that what Sam suggests can be a good idea, especially in the scope of larger social and emotional learning that young people throughout the world could benefit from receiving. Yet as we explored in this book,

---

"Strategies like dissociation can have costs, yet whatever helped you to survive we are grateful for."   —THOMAS ZIMMERMAN

"I'm a funny person in general but my parts are even funnier! I think my brain is awesome. It's helped me come as far as I have today and I have beaten a lot of odds. Having DID isn't a death sentence. You need to respect your brain."   —ALEXIS

"Having many different characters to pull from and say—that's part of me, but that's not all of me. That helps me to reduce shame."

—SUNNEE HOPE

"I wouldn't be alive without dissociation. I'm so appreciative that I was able to create parts, so indebted for the parts that helped me survive."

—OLGA TRUJILLO

while they are an important part of the picture, teaching skills and strategies is only half of the picture. There is a great deal of work that must be done on a systemic and societal level to call out problematic dissociation when we see it being created by these systems.

A major part of that systemic oppression includes the way mental health services operate in the United States and many countries throughout the world. At the time of this writing, so many people in need of high-quality trauma counseling are not able to access it unless they have an ability to pay, especially in places we collectively call community mental health. Additionally, the most highly skilled and trained therapists—which I am sad to say includes me—see getting out of the horrible way that community and other institutional systems can treat therapists as a career goal. We congratulate other therapists for getting out on their own, yet in turn, some of the most vulnerable people can be left without the care they most need. This phenomenon may be the greatest dissociation of all that was created by societies and systems that do not place value on mental health care and treating mental health workers well.

This issue is another place where I may be leaving you with more questions instead of answers, and any answers that are out there are certainly not easy to materialize. Especially when so many of us are trying to function and make a living in systems that are dissociative and oppressive in nature. Yes, it can feel exhausting to work toward dismantling the walls and building the bridges, especially when our instincts tell us that we need to let it all collapse so we can build something more functional and welcoming to all. Doing any

---

"Being able to see from a dissociative state abstractly is part of leadership capacity. But it matters who is in your dissociative states because a lot of lightworkers are non-grounded people who don't have a lot of ancestral scaffolding."   —TADA HOZUMI

"The trauma is what is a burden on my life. What I've been through was inexcusable. That's the burden, that's the part of it that hurts, not the dissociation. As a student of human consciousness, I wonder if this is just another way of being?"   —MELISSA PARKER

"DID folks are our greatest teachers. I got better at treating everything as I got better with treating dissociative clients. They have helped me to better recognize and respond to dissociation in the vast array of trauma-related presentations I encounter in my practice."

—DR. DEBBIE KORN

kind of advocacy work in this modern climate—whether you are advocating for total change or trying to create change in the places where you operate—can make you feel like you are singing into the void.

I truly believe both the personal skills part and the societal change part of this work begin by having conversations. Sam and I often text about what he is learning and observing about dissociation, and I consider it a privilege to have these conversations with him and many of my other friends. When I tell people about my condition, I often lead with, "So what do you know about the word *dissociation* and what it means?" For many outside the field there is little immediate recognition, so I begin to educate. And then from there people can inevitably start to see some of their own patterns and where dissociation plays out in their lives, both adaptively and maladaptively.

What is one conversation you most need to have when you finish this book? Perhaps it is a conversation to obtain greater insight or help into your own condition, and you seek out the services of a therapist or other healing professional. Maybe it's a conversation you need to have with a family member or partner to begin opening a door for further communication about how you operate in the world. You may be someone who has been on the cusp of coming out about your dissociative mind in a more formal way in your profession, on social media, or in public—how can you start that in a singular conversation with a trusted other? And then be open to the possibilities of where it can go....

And finally, perhaps you are in the position of being able to fully advocate using whatever pathways of privilege are available to you. Such advocacy can happen through your social media platforms, blogs, or article writing. Or perhaps you have the motivation to call for change where policy is made. It can start as simply as calling the licensing boards of your profession in your state and country and asking questions about how professionals with dissociative disorders may be treated. Through having such a meeting or conversation, as I did with my state board, you may be in a position to advocate. Maybe you have interest in making contact with politicians who are able to influence mental health and recovery policy, especially as it relates to equitable access to trauma-focused therapeutic services for all people regardless of their ability to pay. All of these options are needed and on the table.

Or perhaps you see a need to start a new conversation altogether, build a new way of doing things in your own profession. My writing this book is a way that I/we responded to that challenge burning within us. It's our love letter to our mind that dances the dance of dissociation with the partner that is life every day. I wanted to create a different book about dissociation featuring various voices as a way to keep new conversations flowing about how we dismantle stigma and create pathways that help, not hinder, people in a very broken world.

Hopefully the conversations started by the book are just the beginning.

And those of us who chose to *sing anyway,* even if it feels like the people in our lives don't want to listen, will find each other.

EXPRESSIVE ARTS PRACTICE: MAKING A GIFT BOX OR GIFT BAG

Presents often come wrapped in beautiful packages or bags that are either festive or ceremonial. In expressive arts therapy, we often encourage people to decorate a box that serves as a container for all the things you'd like to hold that cannot possibly be dealt with at one time. Although you are certainly welcome to engage in this container practice too, for this concluding practice focused on *gifts,* we are going to put a little twist on it.

Think of how you might prepare to give someone else a gift—in a box with a ribbon, with a bag, a sack, or maybe even an envelope. Prepare one of these for yourself and/or your system, being as simple or as decoratively creative as you'd like. As with all of our expressive arts practices, you can let this practice evolve over time. Eventually, take small pieces of paper and begin notating some of the gifts of dissociation you've experienced in your life. If that's too much of a stretch for you to identify right now, start with gifts or positives about yourself and how you handle the world that you are aware of and can presently work with. As with all practices, you are invited to get as creative as you'd like on the pieces of paper. Perhaps drawing images or symbols works better than words. Or if the idea of a gift box or other container doesn't work for you, perhaps making a playlist (either for listening or dancing) that celebrates you feels more organic.

Keep this gift container (or alternative like a playlist) with you. Keep adding to it with new gifts that you identify or are revealed about yourself as you grow in your healing. These gifts do not even have to be limited to your dissociation. Anything about you, including any small victories, can be used. Consider then coming to your gift box during times when you might be feeling low or doubting yourself. Open the gift, again and again, and notice whatever you notice. My wish for you is that you realize what a wonder you and, if applicable, your internal team, really are.

═══QUESTIONS TO ASK MY THERAPIST OR PSYCHIATRIST═══

- Do you believe that there are positive aspects of dissociation?

- What are your approaches or ideas on how we can treat the problems caused by dissociation, while allowing some of the useful skills to remain?

- What if I told you that many other people with dissociative disorders and DID identify being dissociative as a superpower? How does this land for you?

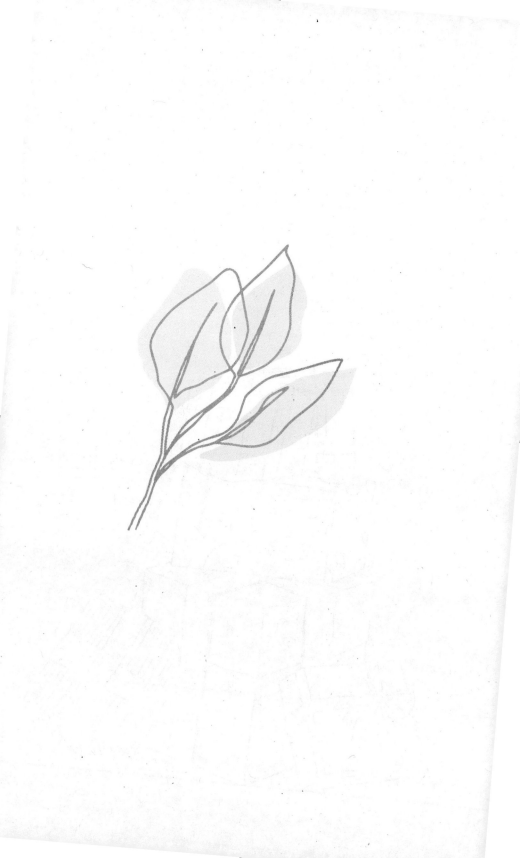

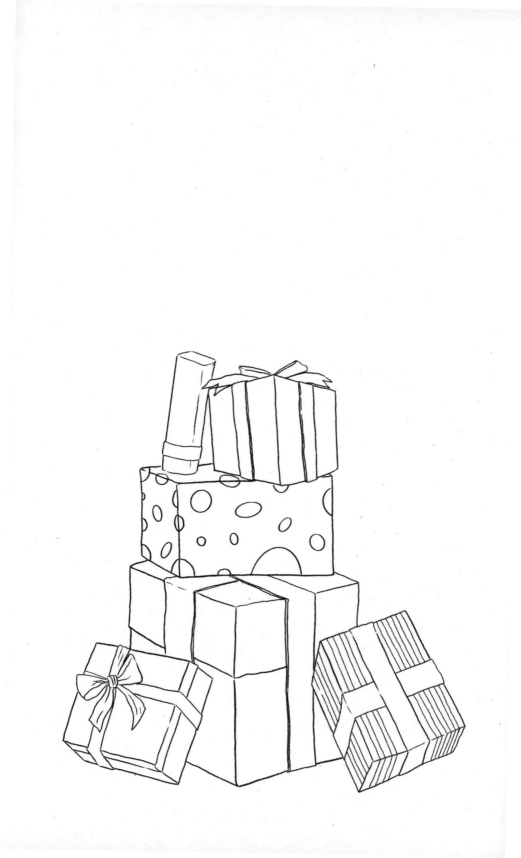

Appendix A

For Clinicians and Therapists

The year was 2006: I literally went running from the first PhD program in Counselor Education that I enrolled in, and *running* is not hyperbole. Myself and my system were overcome with such a sense of "you are not safe here, get out" after meeting with our graduate advisors, our flight mode activated and we went running from the big building at this major state university. Eventually we were able to find a more nontraditional PhD program that celebrated our more prismatic way of seeing the world, and we created work in that program that mainstream journals later published. Yet this experience stayed with me, of just how unsafe people with dissociative minds and other superpowers can feel in institutions. And the people we ran from were entrusted to train the next generation of therapists!

If you are a therapist or other helping professional who has read this book and you are feeling highly unprepared to work with dissociation, the fault is likely not yours. Graduate programs, in my experience, are not preparing students to the degree that they need to for working with trauma and dissociation—if they go there at all. My experience during this first PhD program foreshadowed much of how my career would play out, and I've long existed in the helping professions as an educator who will tell you what you're not going to hear in graduate school. My hope after you read this far is that the material has connected for you on some personal level. Because this is how we take our education and formation as therapists to the next level, to truly be effective in the world where we presently find ourselves.

Remember that we all dissociate, and we all have parts. What have you learned about your Dissociative Profile, as a person, after reading and hopefully working through the book to this point? How can you translate this personal learning to better understand your clients and work more effectively with them? Before reading on, you may consider taking some time to reflect or freewrite on these questions.

Before moving into the heart of the chapters, I invite you to consult the Recommended Reading and Resources section for more information on where you can access some of the scales and strategies referenced in this chapter. In sum, there is much more training available if you believe you need it after reading the book and this Appendix. An Infinite Mind and The International Society for the Study of Trauma and Dissociation (ISSTD) are continuously running trainings and making resources available. In 2021 my own company, The Institute for Creative Mindfulness, launched a special certificate program in dissociative studies for EMDR Therapists, and we hope at some point to expand this to all clinicians. Becoming competent in working with dissociative disorders is about more than just taking technical training and having mastery of scales and interviews, although these can certainly be helpful at the beginning of your clinical endeavors and as valuable continuing education as the field progresses. This Appendix will primarily focus on contributor wisdom, with the understanding that you can continue your inquiry further with the plethora of resources that exist.

The interviews with our contributors revealed several important areas I wish to cover with you in this Appendix. Although this section is primarily written for people who work as clinical professionals, you might also draw benefit if you work professionally in any of the healing or spiritual arts. Moreover, if you are reading this book in the role of client or survivor of trauma who wants to seek help, the content might assist you in further determining what you are looking for in a therapist or other professional. The Appendix is divided into four sections: Professional Voices, Relational Issues, Technical Considerations, and Points of Fusion between Relational Work and Clinical Techniques.

Professional Voices

For Elizabeth Davis, it's important for therapists to get educated about dissociation as a normal experience. She says, "It's about living in the world, not having an abnormal connection to the world." Elizabeth also believes it is important to treat people with dissociative symptoms like everyone else, as making dissociative folks an anomaly is harmful to them. Sandra Johnson echoes this sentiment, observing that the more she hears her colleagues talk about working with dissociation as a specialty, "the worse it gets." For Elizabeth, much of this normalization also involves helping all clients understand their inner parts landscape, even if they don't have dissociative disorders or DID.

Dr. Curt Rounazoin, in reflecting back on his over forty years of treating DID, cautions professionals not to let their chosen paradigms of understanding human behavior blind them to the reality of who and what is sitting in front of them in their offices. To the professionals who say that dissociation—especially DID—doesn't exist, he says that's like believing that trauma doesn't exist. He notes, "It's like you're dealing with the bullet wound and do not believe that the bleeding is part of the wound." Curt also wants other therapists to know that, based on his experience, most of the DID clients he's worked with are highly competent and highly educated, and they show up in almost every profession.

Dr. Debbie Korn believes that screening for dissociation must become a standard part of your clinical practice for every client who walks through your door. The major screening and diagnostic instruments that clinicians have at their disposal are covered in the Recommended Reading and Resources section. She also cautions that sometimes dissociative disorders remain undiagnosed until far into treatment because several of the parts who see themselves as "frontline protectors" might be too invested in keeping the nature of your client's mind hidden. Debbie believes that communicating a message like "all parts are welcome" early into the treatment process is your best chance for helping the system feel more comfortable when the time seems ideal. Communication within the overall safe container of the therapeutic relationship, for Debbie, "is everything." When one of your clients does receive a DID diagnosis, people need to know that it's treatable and in some cases curable.

The anonymous EMDR trainer who contributed to the project says that you have to be able to see complex trauma to treat it, and he believes that this is where many EMDR therapists are lacking in their skills. He continues, "Having your eyes open really makes a difference." All of the voices featured in this section believe that having a repertoire of stabilization strategies and one solid, experiential approach to trauma-focused care (like EMDR Therapy,

Somatic Experiencing, Clinical Hypnosis, Expressive or Creative Arts thera-pies) is crucial for success. Dr. Korn adds, "People only get somewhat better with talk therapy."

Relational Issues

In chapter 6, where we explored options for treatment and healing, the rela-tional imperative emerged as a theme in and of itself as vital to the healing process. While there is recognition that the relationship between the thera-pist and the client can serve as the solid foundation for good therapeutic tech-niques to occur, for most contributors, getting to the helpful techniques would not have happened without the relationship established. In this section we'd like to share with you what some of our contributors offered when asked what they would want helping professionals to know about working with someone like them. These responses specifically address relational elements.

Alexis's sharing on the importance of the therapeutic relationship covers several key points. First, patience is the number one priority. Patience and building trust: "If I don't trust you, I'm not going to talk to you." She also emphasizes the imperative of flexibility, recognizing that it can be a diffi-cult ride to guide someone with DID. "You have to buckle up and be flexible because it's never the same." In reflecting on her own experiences in therapy she says, "I like the fact that I lead therapy and never feel pushed or retrauma-tized myself, even when I sense that my own therapist is two steps ahead of me. I like gentle guidance but when it's completely within my control."

Erin gave unfiltered responses from each major part in her system. Her eight-year-old self said, "Just hang out with us and tell us what you know, let's just explore; go emotional adventuring together; play in the sandbox." Her twelve-year-old part says, "Just know that everyone is different and so cool. That can be fun and scary, but that's what makes life what it is." To therapists everywhere, her sixteen-year-old part says, "Stop putting all of your shit on me and do your own work. Stop being an asshole to people." And all together as her present self, Erin offers, "How can we just show up? Don't be there to fix your client and think that you're some sort of dissociative client whisperer. Just show up. The relationship is most healing, I don't care what modality you are using."

Erin also gets annoyed when she hears fellow professionals say, "I'm scared, what if they decompensate?" She emphasizes, "Trust that they know how to survive. They've survived horrible stuff already. You're there to make it easier." Danielle says very clearly to her fellow therapists, "We can smell your fear a mile away." TaNiya adds, "I know when you're triggered by me." Adam O'Brien words it as, "Know thyself; because I can already see through your game."

Melissa Parker continues, "Use your fear as a guide—but not about your client, about yourself and your system. What is your fear telling you? What is the spot of concern that you have? Is it about your client, or is it about you?" Melissa also adds that it's vital for professionals to recognize that the pathology is there because of the trauma and the abuse, *not* because of the survivor and their system. As a person with DID, Melissa adds, "For us, safety is being able to trust ourselves and our reality; to trust each other (client-to-therapist) and all of the people on the inside." Susan Pease Banitt offers her perspective, "Be willing to enter into my reality with me without deciding what my reality is." She adds that this quality is what makes her current therapist perfect for her even though the therapist isn't specifically trained in trauma work.

Samantha Wagner emphasizes from her perspective as a child that it is important to be loving and caring when you go through this process and work with someone. She remembers, "So many times Mom would read things like 'people with DID are dangerous' and I saw how upset that made her." Samantha encourages therapists everywhere to educate themselves in order to refrain from making broad judgments when working with someone with DID.

Megan reminds us that it can be hard for people to open up about mental health in general—let alone DID—because we can fear being seen as "crazy," so for her, the therapeutic alliance is the most important part of therapy. Kylie also believes that the relationship is most important; to feel that she is with someone who cares, who is listening, and who is present in that moment. As a person of faith, she personally appreciates when a professional is willing to go there with her, and that safety is necessary. "I need to feel safe," she says, "and I just know it when I feel it." For Dianne Harper the safety was created by professionals who were able to help her address some of her practical issues in life, helping her establish structure for herself. She reflects, "There is something about being present with me, where I am; walk with me and hold the grounded space when needed so I don't have to worry about that." In remembering her own therapeutic journey, Dianne remembers one session where her therapist allowed her to just curl up in a ball of pillows and be a scared, hurt, traumatized being.

Jacqueline Lucas adds that therapists need to help clients guide their relationship with dissociation, explaining, "Silence can be so helpful with that and a lot of therapists aren't so helpful with silence as there's a lot of rapid-fire talking and explaining going on in most therapy. It can be hard for clients to process something in thirty seconds." Thomas Zimmerman advises therapists to start by listening. He contends, "It would not have been helpful for me to be run through anyone's program. The first counselor I ever saw just listened, and her presence was a needed container." A.J. believes that the single most important thing you can do for your clients is to listen, and then follow up with a *tell me more*. She adds, "You need to know where your client is going before you can comment on something. And the client may not understand that therapists are trained to and often want to put everything into boxes." Malika says that in her engagement with therapy, she first needed to be heard without any judgment. For her, this connects to the yogic teaching of observation without judgment. She reflects, "I didn't have the capacity to do this at first so I needed someone to model it for me."

Amy Wagner cautions that we can fall into this trap of, "I've seen this before, it's the same." Several other contributors note how unhelpful it felt to be told that they fit some kind of typical profile for PTSD, DID, or any number of issues. Amy goes on, "There is no way to manualize working with someone who experiences complex trauma and a dissociative response. That brings up a big need to be humble and to keep asking questions." Katharine said that even though she agrees that being pigeonholed into a diagnostic profile isn't helpful, she did have a fear that she was the only one who struggled with these things. So as a therapist, being able to navigate the line between validating and normalizing—while also being open to asking questions and not seeing your clients through a textbook lens—is critical.

We believe that using a rigid textbook understanding of anything connected to dissociation is impractical. Kathleen said very bluntly, "Trash the formula. Work with the person and not the formula." Dr. Kirsten Koenig said that to work with her, one must "throw out the textbook." In speaking to the importance of authenticity in the therapeutic relationship, Heather (LS) Scarboro+ notes, "Set the intervention-based book aside. Set it aside, that's not who you are looking at. You are looking at a body with many body bus drivers. You are working with a person who has many persons, and there are many ears listening to you."

While there is nothing necessarily wrong with having textbook knowledge and studying about dissociation, for Christy Dunn it's about acknowledging that the client has the most information about their lived experience, not you. Christy sees that approaching therapy as your client's equal and not their expert is vital to maintaining cultural humility and competent care. Michelle Kahl adds that it's important for therapists to see the person beyond the diagnosis. BeeJay says: "You have educational expertise but they have the most expertise about themselves. When someone comes out to you as DID, keep your biases aside, open your mind, and just meet somebody where they are."

Blaise reflects back on the mixed messages he received during his own graduate training: Build rapport, yet be a robot. He remembers getting feedback that he was too relaxed in sessions and people wouldn't take him seriously. What stung even more is that the feedback came from a Black male professor. Yet Blaise has learned throughout his young career that people seem to like him and connect with him because he is real, and that's a quality he also looks for in a therapist who might be working with him.

An issue that comes up often when working with highly traumatized clients with unhealed attachment wounds is how to establish and negotiate boundaries. Many of our contributors experienced issues with previous therapists who tried to be everything for them—therapist, parent, friend—and that ended up causing more damage. The generally accepted wisdom is to establish firmer boundaries at the beginning with all clients, letting them know what you can or can't do as their therapist. Yet Katarina Lundgren speaks to the importance of transparency and consistency. An example of transparency is letting your clients know early on what you are not willing to do, yet also having a willingness to explore and to negotiate. She offers this example, "If a client wanted to go out for ice cream, explore it and what it would mean to the relationship before outright saying no." Katarina says that practicing true curiosity, empathy, and compassion in a nonjudgmental way is crucial because the power imbalances in therapy can be problematic for the client since part of therapy can involve them handing over their power to you as the therapist.

Crystal offers some very specific guidance to therapists, which must first start with listening. "Don't come in and sound like a recording or like you're reading a book in your head," she cautions. "I'm not a book. Don't come in with preconceived ideas. There is no science to this."

Her second piece of advice is to be able to offer comfort and validate. And if you can't handle it, she believes, step out of the way and communicate this authentically. She also feels that therapist–patient role rigidity is unnecessary, yet boundaries can still be present even when rigidity is not. For example, Crystal feels very strongly that appropriate therapeutic touch can be important.

Crystal says that when she's curled up on the floor crying, "That's me as a child sitting there. There are ways to offer that child comfort that may involve a hug or a touch." She believes that there are ways to engage touch without crossing a line, perhaps having a discussion up front about rules of engagement around touch. For example, a good alternative for her even if a person is comfortable hugging her is to sit back-to-back with them. In this way she feels the physical support but there might not be the awkwardness of intimacy that she knows some clients may experience.

A final issue to cover is an area where dissociative specialists can be of split opinion—how to work with the younger parts, sometimes called "the littles." Some therapists believe it's most important to talk to an adult client as an adult, yet be mindful that there are younger parts inside who may need things broken down. Cheryl, who has DID, likes to be worked with in this way, saying, "As much as we have child parts, we're not children. Don't talk to us or treat us like children. We're adults, we're whole people, we have feelings; we need to sort out what's going on."

The Garden System, another contributor with DID, believes differently. Also remember that The Garden System does not identify a sole host or core part, so the necessity of a professional talking to one of her littles may take on more meaning. She shared with us as a postscript to her interview:

> We noticed that there is very little information out there on how to handle someone's littles. Pretty much, they are always told to tuck away. The only article that I found that addressed littles basically said not to treat them like real children. While it said what not to do, it didn't say what to do. We hear that a lot of therapists don't want to talk to the littles or address them or work with them. Which we think is really sad because they are the ones that hold the trauma and need the most help in our opinion. Our current therapist is very welcoming of whoever comes to session. And when we started talking with you [Jamie], you didn't make a big deal that it was Jenny out talking to you. In a way, when our littles feel acknowledged and when Jenny feels that it is okay for her to be out, then she is more willing to let the others out to talk. Therapists should not be afraid to talk to parts that are not "the host" or parts that are little. We believe if a part is out, there is a reason they are out.

In contrasting Cheryl's and The Garden System's sharing, it reminds me once more that there are no hard and set rules for working with DID or dissociation. As guided by many of our contributors in this section, you have to be willing to be flexible, meet a client and their system where they are at, and build the treatment plan accordingly. Be open to what they have to share with you on relational preference. In doing that, you would, for example, have two different ways of operating if Cheryl and The Garden System were both your clients.

Technical Considerations

Although our contributors emphasized the importance of the therapeutic relationship as a main point of emphasis, many of our contributors also answered our open-ended question about what they would say to helpers about some elements of technique, training, and competence. Jaime Pollack of An Infinite Mind recognizes that every professional needs to start somewhere on their journey of becoming more competent in working with dissociation, but don't try to figure it out on your own. She states, "Reading one book or taking one class can make you DID aware, but it does not make you DID competent. Supervision and consultation is needed to help you navigate it. Find another professional who has been down the road and through the swamp. Get a guide so you don't get eaten by the monsters."

Paula S. agrees. She comments,

> In our profession, we are thrust into our roles way too soon without enough quality supervision and mentorship—we are flung into a traumatic box where we are overworked right away. We almost have to dissociate from our own experiences as a therapist. CBT can assist with that—managing feelings that we are inadequate, feeling that we have to brainwash ourselves into feeling that what we're doing is enough. We're not imposters, but it's possible that we're doing harm and not doing enough until we educate ourselves and do our own work. I personally had to remortgage my house to finance my further training and doing my own therapeutic work. The whole system is messed up.

One of our anonymous contributors shares in great detail some of the technical considerations that she would like to see enacted in clinical services. She says,

> I never got the dissociative disorder diagnosis until 2019 because nobody looked! I think that the Dissociative Experiences Scale (DES) should be some kind of standard screening that they give you in hospitals or residential settings. I was "high functioning," but that should have been a clue for them to look deeper. I had pains in my body and that should have been a clue. My body had such an ill reaction to EMDR Therapy and diving into my deep trauma, that should have been a clue. If you do have a clue and treating these things is not in your skill set, then send to a colleague for further assessment.

sunnEe hope believes that therapists ought to be trained to look for the subtle signs of dissociation—changes in facial expression, body language, changes in voice, when people become nonresponsive or change into some younger version of themselves. She adds, "Have compassion for however the person presents themselves. If someone begins to change the way they are presenting, give them space, don't press louder, faster, and harder." Helping the person who is experiencing dissociation to recognize and befriend it is also vital, in her view.

Rebecca adds that being both trauma- and addiction-informed in your therapeutic work is critical. She also sees the importance of educating clients on what to expect with various forms of treatment you might try and keeping an openness to feedback at any time in the spirit of collaboration. John Fugett says quite plainly, "Therapists need to be trauma-informed. Any therapist who does not get specific trauma training should not be seeing anyone. If my early psychiatrists and therapists would have known how to ask about early childhood trauma, it would have saved me decades. But I sense they were caught up in the fear around false memories." Andrea concurs that it is important to be trauma-informed and to assess for trauma. She adds that one time a therapist told her, "You don't have PTSD," and said therapist never asked her a single question about her childhood! Andrea says that although it is important to assess for trauma, it's okay if you don't get someone's full story on the first day. She continues, "Let what they disclose evolve over time, yet let them know that you are open about what they have to say."

Holli Ellis shares with great emphasis, *"Our bodies matter.* Integrating the body and the mind is imperative in treatment. Educate the people you are working with and give them the tools for how to tend to their bodies and how to exist in their bodies." Jackson explains three tasks that he sees as vital: (1) regulate, using any ways that you know how to regulate the clients (e.g., breathing, yoga, other resourcing), (2) relate, (3) rationalize, or put things into perspective for your client. Julian Jaramillo challenges fellow therapists to "devote yourselves to honing the ability to let the native, the organic wisdom of each client to emerge."

In addition to some of the basics, like not telling your clients they are in a "safe space" and being mindful of commands like "get into a comfortable position," Chuck Bernsohn cautions that many therapists lack nuanced understanding around dysphoria, especially as it shows up with trans people. Chuck advises, "Notice how you talk to someone about their body. For example, if you are guiding EMDR self-tapping, listen to how a person talks about their body and then deliver the cues and directives accordingly." Language matters and working in collaboration with the client on how they regard their bodies is important. Destiny Aspen Mowadeng emphasizes the importance of inclusion. She notes,

> What you put on the website is not enough, saying you're inclusive. There are so many other factors to consider. With learning disabilities, find out what is the best way that a person takes in information. Be mindful that not all places in the world have disability access laws. Be mindful that not emailing your clients back can be a barrier to clients who rely heavily on text-based communication. Be mindful of the impact of caretakers. Being truly inclusive with disability takes hard work.

Destiny also wants people to know that both disabled individuals and survivors of complex trauma use dark humor as a coping mechanism. She adds, "I ask all the time—am I human or am I cyborg? There is so much metal in me!" She also wants professionals to know that suicidal thinking can be incredibly common for people with disabilities and complex trauma. Knowing how to handle it in a way that doesn't shame your client is essential. Destiny advises use of the questions, "What are the feelings behind it? What the hell is driving it?" She recognizes, and I concur, that knowing the legal parameters in your place of practice are important, yet so much suicidal ideation can really come from a part or aspect of experience needing to be heard. In our experience, the same phenomenon can apply to non-suicidal self-injury.

Safety planning and assessing for risk to self or others is an issue of great concern to many therapists. We are all trained to be aware of the legalities and ethics in the states and countries where we practice. While it is not my intention to override the guidelines where you practice, I also advise you to be competent in what provisions are in place where you practice for keeping clients out of psychiatric hospitals wherever possible. Since the beginning of my professional work with dissociation, I've strongly articulated my beliefs that an inpatient psychiatric facility can be one of the least safe places for a person who dissociates—especially if the presence of their dissociation or DID is negated by the treating staff. I've formed this clinical opinion largely from seeing how my clients who dissociated have been treated in mainstream psychiatric facilities, and my lived experience doing everything in my power to stay safe when I've been in a suicidal or self-injurious mode—except going to the hospital. My plan usually involves leaning strongly into my support system, taking some time to rest, and contacting my therapist. I know inherently, as The Garden System reported in their interview, that a traditional psychiatric facility would be a dehumanizing place for me. And there are only a select few, in the United States at least, that are specifically dissociation-competent. While there are some movements toward making inpatient care more trauma-informed, we have a long way to go.

If you are a professional and have concerns about normalizing ideation around harm to self or others, which can include suicidal ideation, please seek supervision or consultation for navigating these issues with clients who dissociate. I've long observed that people are hesitant to articulate their struggles because they are afraid they will be hospitalized, yet having a therapeutic space where people feel safe enough to name them when they are happening is vital. In my experience, naming them and having the chance to identify how they may connect to the system's larger issues can defuse a great deal of their power. Of course you will need to identify and review protective factors, and be mindful of any additional steps you might need to take if what a client articulates is at the level of intent or plan. Yet as a professional culture we must defuse our own fears about working with client struggles around suicidal ideation or ideation of other harm to self or others.

There are many more calls from contributors emphasizing the need to work with the whole person, not just treat them with psychiatric drugs. Paula also emphasizes that many professionals think they have to get an entire trauma narrative to work well with trauma, but that is not the case. By having a solid relational foundation and good set of embodied skills, you can recognize that trauma is a struggle for someone and plan treatment accordingly without going into excessive detail in your questioning. Dr. Kellie Kirksey believes that really exploring with clients what has worked for them in the past to make them feel good is critical in what she calls "rehydrating" and "reengaging" them. Connecting to breath and visualization can widen a client's ability to contain in her estimation, so having skills of this nature to share are essential. She says it's important to be a student of the client's own reality, which she defines as a personal belief of what is true in the moment.

Points of Fusion between Relational Work and Clinical Techniques

A quality therapeutic experience requires a fusion between solid relational skills and appropriate implementation of clinical techniques. Several of our contributors spoke to this idea directly in their reflections. For Fiona, success comes down to four primary elements:

- As a therapist, look at your own dissociation; do your own work before attempting to do mine.

- Get a rapport: how present are you? If you're disconnected and can't put your finger on why, take the risk to name it and to check it (under your own supervision or, if appropriate, with your client).

- Disregard everything you think you know about dissociation before meeting me, and *really* meet me; even the good stuff you've learned, wear it like a very loose cloak.

- Obtain some type of training to recognize the subtle dissociation as it presents in the room, which includes being able to track when someone isn't fully present.

Although other items mentioned in this Appendix add more of the specifics of what you as a therapist may need to address, Fiona's list provides a solid overview.

Since many professionals ask what screenings, scales, or clinical interviews they ought to be giving to assess for the presence of clinically significant dissociation, we do want to share one cautionary tale that emerged here from the interviews. Every contributor who advocated for the use of screenings mentioned the Dissociative Experiences Scale (DES), a twenty-eight-item inventory developed by Eva Carlson and Frank Putnam that asks some common questions about dissociative experiences (e.g., some people have the experience of driving or riding in a car or bus or subway and suddenly realizing they don't remember what happened during all or part of the trip). People are then asked to rank what percentage of the time that experience happens to them, and an average score above certain numbers may reveal the presence of a dissociative disorder. The DES, available as an adult and adolescent version, is a screen and not a diagnostic inventory, so a full clinical interview would need to be given to confirm the diagnosis. For clinicians needing a formal method other than their own interviewing strategies, the Structured Clinical Interview for Dissociative Disorders (SCID-D) is most commonly used and most highly validated.[1]

In recent years, the Multidimensional Inventory of Dissociation (MID), developed by Paul Dell, has become more popular in trauma-focused circles. Also featuring both an adult and adolescent version, the MID contains 218 questions that can assist professionals in arriving at a diagnosis and points of analysis that might form the treatment. As a client, I found taking the MID to be an exhausting and confusing process—all of my parts wanted to answer each question differently and the entire exercise felt far too linear to even begin to capture what was going on with me. I do not use the MID or any instruments that might cause more stress for my clients unless I am totally stumped on a diagnostic picture. Because training you receive on dissociation might advocate for use of the MID, I wanted to make sure to at least mention it in this Appendix, and feature the experience of our one contributor who shared how it was used in her treatment.

Amy Wagner said that when her therapist gave her the MID, it was not the MID itself that proved problematic for her; it was her therapist's reaction to her MID score. Amy says, "The MID was actually a confirming experience for me. But then I saw the blood run out of my therapist's face when she saw how high the score was. That was the traumatic part." Amy believes something that I have long taught: let any of these inventories be something that starts or furthers conversation with your clients, not something that you get hung up on scoring. Know that these inventories can let the client feel more validated in their experiences, but as a clinician, do not get too caught up on assigning meaning to a number. Like many principles of relationship discussed throughout the book, listening is most important. So let the inventories promote more conversation that will help you further understand the client's inner world.

Alicia Hann offered a story from one of her treatment episodes that serves as a powerful cautionary tale to all of us, about how what therapists think might be helpful in addressing dissociation actually reflects a lack of understanding about dissociation. Her therapist noticed that she lost time during her purging episodes, and he suspected that the response was dissociative. But that was about the only thing he got right. After that, he instructed her to get a foghorn and put it in the bathroom. His intention was for her to blow the foghorn whenever she needed to "wake up," yet Alicia explains that "all it did was announce the shame." She summarized, "It wasn't pleasant."

Alicia is not the only contributor to this volume who has a horror story about well-intentioned interventions that went horribly wrong. Yet her emphasis on the line "all it did was announce the shame" encapsulates so much of why clients who dissociate can struggle. The most impactful definition of shame I use in my work is attributed to the French–Cuban feminist author Anaïs Nin: "Shame is the lie that someone told you about yourself." Although this quote of hers is often placed on memes and posters, perhaps another of her teachings ought to ring even more powerfully with the solution for healing shame:

> The truth, which only the child and the artist tell, is the real wonder. Magic and power lie in the truth, the truth.[2]

As therapists or other helping professionals, we must recognize that in some way, we are in a position of power—even if our intention is to immediately become collaborative. In a position of power, we can either reinforce messages of shame—which can include that people are somehow defective for even dissociating in the first place, or we can help people see new truths about themselves.

What is one new truth that you might help one of your clients who dissociates to see about themselves after learning what you've learned in this book?

Maybe there are several—take some time at the end of this Appendix to reflect on this question, either via writing or some other form of meditation or contemplation.

Appendix B

For Loved Ones, Friends, and Connections of People with Dissociative Disorders and Complex Trauma

I am writing *Dissociation Made Simple* at the beginning of an exciting new romantic relationship in my personal life. Regardless of how this adventure may unfold in the future, my/our partner has already given us one of the most loving gifts—the space to talk openly and honestly about our dissociative disorder. This is scary new territory, even for me. In my two previous marriages and other romantic relationships, it was always easier to say that I had PTSD. Eventually, discussion about parts of experience would come out, and eventually the "D" word would enter the conversation. Yet the idea of leading with, "Hi, my name is Jamie and I have a dissociative disorder . . ." then having to break down the explanation felt like I was just setting myself up for rejection before the would-be partner even had a chance to know me. Of course this can feel dishonest, yet it speaks to the reality that still abounds in mainstream culture—that PTSD can carry less stigma than dissociative disorders even though both are rooted in trauma.

Our contributor Alexis calls disclosing your DID or other dissociative disorders "dropping the DID bomb," and one of the trickiest issues for people with dissociative disorders can be negotiating the timing if they enter a relationship knowing that they have them. If we disclose them at the beginning we might scare people, and not just romantic partners—coworkers, friends, other people in the community—the stigma might prevent people from seeing beyond our condition. Yet if we wait to disclose dissociation should we need to, it can feel like we are lying. Over the years I've treated many people who chose not to be fully transparent with their partners or other family members about their DID or other trauma-based conditions, fearing the judgment and misunderstanding even in some cases where partners are loving and kind. Our protective parts can help us keep the secret, yet holding back the ocean (metaphorically speaking) can come with its own level of strain on a person and their system.

I felt it important to include this Appendix in *Dissociation Made Simple* because many people with dissociative disorders struggle not only with explaining the way their mind works to others, we can also struggle with interpersonal effectiveness in general. Our various parts might be easily triggered or have serious opinions about how people treat us and how we treat other people. Yet many of us have chosen to live a full and interactive life with others despite having been wounded by people. There can be so many more partners to dance with as we navigate this dance of dissociation on the shaky floor of life that we introduced in chapter 1.

Many people I generally refer to as loved ones, friends, and connections—spouses, partners, parents, children, friends, and even coworkers and members of the community—are seeking genuine understanding and want to know how they can best support the people in their lives who struggle with dissociation. In this Appendix, I sometimes refer to you collectively as "trusted others." My hope is that you have read the book and worked through some of the exercises to gain a better understanding of those you care about, and see where trauma and dissociation may show up in your life. You may already be realizing that you are not so different from those you care about, after all. This Appendix features many of our contributors sharing in the interviews what they most wanted others to know about navigating life with people like them. We've generally organized this Appendix into the themes that emerged from this sharing—the importance of educating yourself as a trusted other, the imperative of validating and asking the appropriate questions, and how to be helpful with grounding and regulating. Various types of relationships and connections are covered in some of the contributions, and you are encouraged to take what might fit for you in your situation. The contributors also spoke to the necessity of making sure you take care of yourselves and your mental health as you navigate life with a person who has a dissociative mind. Please consider this guidance to be a given as you read through the rest of this Appendix. We hope that some of the exercises and strategies provided in this book have already or will prove helpful to this process.

Before moving into the sections I want to recognize that some of you may feel ready and willing to do these things; and some of you may feel like your loved one, friend, or connection has "the problem" so all of this is on them to sort out. Even as professionals we must make judgment calls on whether spouses, parents, children, and others in a family system are safe enough people to engage in the work. We certainly hope that if you are reading the book and have stuck with us up to this point, you qualify as the latter. None of what we are presenting here ought to be taken as justification to further shame or belittle the person in your life who may have a dissociative experience of life. We present this information in good faith that you have their best interests at heart.

Educating Yourself as a Trusted Other

The more you learn about dissociative responses, the better position you might be in to help the person in your life. Dr. Debbie Korn says that in her practice she educates family members or partners on dissociation, which includes recommended reading, in the same way she educates her clients. Part of dissociation is that the person in question may not recognize how their behaviors look to others, so family, friends, or trusted others helping them to begin identifying their early warning signs can aid the healing process. Debbie recognizes that every person is different in terms of what they want others in their life to know about their internal system and what might work for them in the way of boundaries (e.g., is it okay for the trusted other to call a person's therapist if needed, and if so, when?). To again emphasize the importance of honorable intentions, a loved one, friend, or connection educating themselves on dissociation must never take advantage of or manipulate a person when they are in dissociative responses. I personally, and our contributors, cannot emphasize this enough.

Jaime Pollack encourages loved ones, friends, and connections to get information so that you can understand what your loved one is going through and why they are acting the way they are. She also encourages that trusted others get support for themselves in this process, noting, "Your feelings are legitimate and it's important for you to have an outlet too." An Infinite Mind, the organization founded by Jaime, has specific information available for loved ones and a special track for loved ones at their Healing Together conference.

Christy Dunn also stresses the importance of educating yourself about dissociation in the context of doing your own work as a loved one, friend, or connection. She acknowledges that there is complexity in dissociative experiences and that all of this can be confusing to a loved one. Christy continues, "The more that you are able to be patient, empathetic, and understanding, you will be able to genuinely listen and be attuned. And the better things will work out."

Validating and Asking Appropriate Questions

Alexis wants you, regardless of your role, to know that when someone opens up to you about their DID or other dissociative disorder, they are placing a great deal of trust in you. She underscores the importance of patience and trusting the process, declaring that understanding is not something that will happen overnight. "It's going to take time," she said.

In reflecting back on what helped her in her healing journey, Amy Wagner sang the praises of her daughter Samantha as being the one member of her nuclear family unit who never dishonored any of her parts. Amy said quite simply, "Sam knew how to show up for me." In my interview with Samantha (Sam), she shared, "I just wanted to be there for my Mom. I read things that she asked me to, and helped her out when I could. It was easy for me because I didn't have any preconceived notions of DID. I maintain that I grew up with a loving mom and also that something is wrong here. I took on an attitude of, *what can I do to help?*"

Not everyone who shares about their DID or other dissociative disorders has such a beautiful experience. Dianne Harper, who believes that the best thing trusted others can do is to be present for the people they care about, states that she has not shared her diagnosis with much of her family because she knows they are not safe to share it with. She explains that she had to cut herself off from much of her family for years because they weren't safe for her or for her own child. When she attempted to tell her own child about her history close to three years ago, he put up a wall about not wanting to hear it. She said that this was a huge sadness for her and she is still unsure how she wants to navigate it. She also reports telling a few of her close friends about her story and her experience with DID and lost two of them over it, so she's refrained from speaking about it with other friends, which she says is hard. Her longtime romantic partner of five years, who is now deceased, knew about her dissociative mind—she said that she did not feel good about being in a committed relationship with him if she didn't disclose it. She said that he was fine with it overall and had a knack for asking really good questions like, "Where are you at *now* with all of this?" Dianne concludes, "When someone takes that first little step of telling you, believe them and follow through."

The Garden System discloses that it's been a struggle to get their parents to understand them. Their mother believes that when they go to the hospital or to treatment it's for a vacation, and they recently said to their father, "You don't understand because you don't want to." They wish that their parents would understand that there are going to be days they are capable of doing a lot of things and taking on a lot of responsibility, and there will be days when they don't want to come out. There will be days when they can function like a "normal," healthy adult, and there will be times when they can't. They add, "It's okay to feel feelings other than happiness, and sometimes it's okay to just sit with our feelings. It's okay to just be who we are."

Heather (LS) Scarboro+ realizes that their case is not typical, having been constantly surrounded by validating family members and friends. Their own spouse also has DID and LS+ describes their life together as fun. Sometimes their younger parts or littles have playdates with each other and holiday time can be very interesting as different parts get different gifts for each other from the likes of Santa Claus. To all partners and trusted others Heather (LS+) advises, "Suspend your disbelief. Disbelieving is re-traumatization and this is not helpful as we are trying to build healthy, natural supports."

Alicia Hann recognizes that presence is important from family members and trusted others, as is being nonjudgmental. Having permission to talk, using the language of parts, with others is also helpful for her. As it relates to her eating disorder recovery, she encourages others to refrain from making comments about food or weight. She's noticed that family members can be fixated on *fixing* their loved one, and she advises, "Trust that even mid-struggle, people are doing the best that they can." Sarah Smith says, "Even though it's important not to be in denial about behaviors that you might observe, trust that your person is still a whole person. You may be seeing different parts or different aspects of the person if their actions are troubling you or puzzling you. Please keep as open of a mind as possible."

Paula offered a piece of lived experience she'd like to share specifically with coworkers and colleagues. She says, "Sometimes you will say things to me and it appears that I digested it, but later on when I go recall it I'm not going to remember it. So please, show me some grace." Paula also recognizes, and this is an experience with which my system personally relates, that when she is having a business conversation she is "on." When the conversation shifts to something more general, she is not. Paula's comments on this phenomenon during her interview allowed us to make a very impactful connection—often when we are in a space where we go back and forth between the professional and the personal (e.g., having a business lunch with someone and we might share some personal connection), information on either might not stay retained. This realization has helped us take the practical action of minimizing business meetings in restaurants where noise can be hard to filter, or keeping more separation between professional business and personal matters in conversations with people.

In reflecting on what she identifies as a successful long-term romantic partnership, Sandra Johnson says that her beloved has a relationship with every single one of her selves. He has been kind and nurturing to the young ones, he has been validating and humorous with those selves who may operate in a certain way. He has been flexible, and Sandra believes that this flexibility is the key. She reflects, "If you have someone who is multiple in your family, know that if the selves want to get to know you, be willing. If not, be okay with that too."

Jacqueline Lucas advocates for giving people in your life the "most generous interpretation of their behaviors." She also recognizes the importance of balance in interactions, commenting, "People can be so afraid to trigger something that they don't do that thing anymore and that's not necessarily helpful. The most helpful thing is to be yourselves in a kind and sweet way, but don't treat your loved one with kid gloves either. We need to give people chances to work through their triggers." Noting the importance of taking breaks or time-outs from interactions and being able to walk away, Jacqueline emphasizes that resetting and touching base at a different time when there is no conflict might be most helpful and useful. In our lived experience, this advice is helpful regardless of the relational connection and can work wonders in romantic relationships, raising children, negotiating family relationships, and managing conflict and discipline in work settings.

Being Helpful with Grounding and Regulating

sunnEe Hope gives the same advice to loved ones, friends, and connections that she gives to therapists: "If someone begins to change the way that they are presenting, give them space. Don't press louder, faster, and harder. Give them space while also finding a way to let them know that you are still there." Rebecca reports that she and her husband have been on a long journey together over the last ten years. If Rebecca expresses to him that she is in a "trauma flare," she asks him to respect her requests for calmness and quiet. She also lets him know that if she needs to keep to herself more, it has nothing to do with him—rather, she is attempting to regulate her nervous system. She continues, "He knows that there may or may not be a time for more details. It does not mean that I love you any less."

Rachael says that her wife was essential in helping her to realize when she "went away." To partners, Rachael offers, "Pay close attention and you may notice that your partner or self isn't their full self or their same self. Also, be gentle, not barging in with 'what the fuck is wrong with you?!?' Curiosity and gentleness is the way. 'Do you feel comfortable telling me why one time you seem one way and the other time you seem another way?'" Rachael also wants partners to know that all the parts who may show up are still your partner. Be open to whatever that part may have to share; she recognizes that this can be disconcerting when you're in an adult relationship. But if you understand what's happening, it can make a lot more sense and allow for a deeper level of understanding in the relationship.

Holli Ellis wants partners and loved ones to know that, although it may be hard work, please do not take things personally. She continues, "Most of the time when we are activated in the present, we are reliving something that happened in the past." For trusted others, she suggests a question like, "What's going on with you right now . . . what is the story that you are telling yourself?" (inspired by the work of Brené Brown). She believes that such an approach can help end the secrets and silence that might be tapping into core shame for the person who is struggling. Meeting those secrets from a place of nonjudgment can help neutralize the shame. TaNiya adds that in order for partners and loved ones not to take things so personally, the best thing they can do is to work on loving themselves. She adds that people with dissociative disorders must also show compassion to their loved ones and trusted others, recognizing that it might not be so easy for them to change so many of their perspectives all at once.

Megan, who also notes the importance of unconditional love and acceptance of people in your life with DID, does recognize that some of her more destructive parts can be difficult for trusted others to handle or address. Megan reflects on having to do a great deal of communication with a friend after one of the more destructive parts went off on said friend. "There was a lot of *I'm sorry* on my end. It can be challenging because it's often for things that I don't remember doing." To the loved one in question like her friend, she also emphasizes the importance of not taking things personally while also being open to debriefing conversations that might help the person (like Megan) and their system navigate what they might need to in order to learn and grow from the experience.

Fiona does not believe it's reasonable to ask a partner or family member to master all of the finesse of what a dissociative person may need to ground or to regulate, yet she does feel it's important for them to know the basics. She believes that romantic partners especially ought to work on this together. Fiona and her partner both struggle with dissociation, so they will engage in a strategy where they squeeze each other's hands to simply stay connected and notice whatever grounding might come. In these situations Fiona says that saying, "I'm here with you" is helpful. She also finds it important for partners to establish a good shared vocabulary, especially if one is able to recognize signs that their partner is in a flashback or other dissociative response. She notes that a simple question like, "Are you dissociating?" can invite a connection back. Fiona feels that engaging in this way can be critical for the partner as well—who may be feeling upset, abandoned, or confused when their loved one is in a dissociative response.

Katharine contends that it's important to let your person who struggles with dissociative responses tell you what they need, reminding us all that people with DID and other dissociative disorders are typically very intelligent. Katharine continues, "Dissociation is such a gift that helped me to survive. To make me feel like it's wrong shuts me down so fast." To partners especially, she encourages you to ask your dissociative loved one how you can most be helpful when they are dissociating or otherwise activated. She says, "Sometimes the answer can be something as simple as *paint with me . . . play with me.*" Katharine encourages you as a partner to join them in their process unless they specifically indicate to you that they need to be left alone.

Jaime Pollack articulates that there are mixed opinions on how much a partner or other loved ones and connections ought to know about the specific parts. This area is very gray and must be negotiated on a case-by-case basis. For instance, although Jaime's husband knows a lot about her condition and her triggers, she's chosen not to let him in on certain details about her system. She notes that in being supportive to your partner or other loved ones, it's often the little things that can carry the greatest weight. Jaime says, "Respect, safety, and boundaries. Like my husband Ruperto knows never to walk in the bathroom when I am in the shower and to let me know before he turns on the blender." Kylie says that in her experience, "I need to feel a certain way. I need to be a certain way. Give me the space to authentically show up with how I am feeling. Let me know that it's okay for me to show up in whatever emotional state that I am in." Kylie adds that she fears not having this in a long-term relationship or connection.

Erin believes that we ought to treat all of our relationships as if the person we are in relationship with (regardless of its form) has complex trauma. This attitude will create that space for intentional support while also allowing everyone involved to set very clear boundaries. She continues, "Everybody has to be doing their own work constantly. And know that your presence can be very healing. You can be grounding when they are dissociating. But also recognize that your partner's whole system may not like you, especially at first. Yet your continued willingness to communicate with your partner and their system will help over time."

I've thought long and hard about what I/we as Jamie would like to say to trusted others as we formally close *Dissociation Made Simple*, the book. In addition to echoing everything our contributors shared through their interviews, we feel safest to share the most vulnerably with people who are also willing to be vulnerable with us. When people don't make us feel like the identified problem or the crazy one, we will engage and put in the hard work for our relationship—in whatever form it might take—to work well. And we certainly appreciate when people take the time to understand that we might need certain accommodations or tasks to regulate, to ground, and to reset. I appreciate when my friends and coworkers, including Erin, can do this for us in professional settings just as I value when my partner and friends can allow for these acts of love in our personal life. Speaking for our system, when trusted others can do that for us, we are all too happy to return the favor for them when they may need a little extra help to navigate their stressors and triggers.

> When we choose to love we choose to move against fear, against alienation and separation. The choice to love is a choice to connect, to find ourselves in the other.
>
> —bell hooks

Recommended Reading and Resources

Many of the resources that appear here are standards I suggest both to professionals I train and those in the general public who might want to learn more about dissociation. In keeping with the spirit of this book, I also gave our contributors a chance to share the resources that they most recommend to you for expanding your education and discovery.

Organizations

An Infinite Mind: www.aninfinitemind.com
The Institute for Creative Mindfulness: www.instituteforcreativemindfulness.com
International Society for the Study of Trauma and Dissociation: www.isst-d.org
Spiritual Directors International: www.sdicompanions.org

Websites, Blogs, and Other Tools

Adrian Fletcher, PsyD: www.drfletch.com
Angeles Arrien, PhD: www.angelesarrien.com
Beauty After Bruises: www.beautyafterbruises.org
Bethany Brand, PhD: https://bethanybrand.com
Carolyn Spring: www.carolynspring.com
DID Research: www.did-research.org
DID Self-Help: www.didselfhelp.com
Discovering DID (K.D. Roche): https://blog.discoveringdid.com
Discussing Dissociation: www.discussingdissociation.com
Dissociative Disorders Interview Schedule: www.rossinst.com/ddis
Dissociative Experiences Scale II: http://traumadissociation.com/des
Fireweed Collective: https://fireweedcollective.org

Fraser's Table: https://connect.springerpub.com/content
/sgremdr/6/4/179?implicit-login=true
Guided Healing Psychology Resources (including DID Emergency Cards):
www.guidedhealingpsychology.com/resources
The Hearing Voices Network: www.hearing-voices.org
The Institute for Creative Mindfulness Dissociation & Addiction Resources: www
.instituteforcreativemindfulness.com/dissociation-addiction-resources.html
Jamie Marich, PhD: www.jamiemarich.com
Jean Houston, PhD: www.jeanhouston.com/Jean-Houston
Judith Orloff, MD: https://drjudithorloff.com
Kristin Neff, PhD: https://self-compassion.org
L.B. Lee: http://healthymultiplicity.com/loonybrain/InfoHome.html
Lissa Rankin, MD: https://lissarankin.com
Michael Harner, PhD: www.shamanism.org
Mindfreedom International: https://mindfreedom.org
Multidimensional Interview of Dissociation (MID): www.mid-assessment.com
Olga Trujillo, J.D: www.olgatrujillo.com
Pandora's Project: https://pandys.org
Privilege as Dissociation (Tada Hozumi): www.youtube.com/watch?v=errSkfnZBbE
The Plural Association: https://thepluralassociation.org
Ritual Abuse, Ritual Crime & Healing: http://ra-info.org
Sidran Institute: www.sidran.org
Structured Clinical Interview for Dissociative Disorders (SCID-D): www.rossinst
.com/Downloads/DDIS-DSM-5.pdf
Teach Trauma: https://teachtrauma.com
Top DD Studies: https://topddstudy.com
Trauma and Dissociative Disorders Explained: http://traumadissociation.com
/index.html
Trauma Made Simple (Dr. Jamie Marich's Resources Website): www.trauma
madesimple.com
Treatment Guidelines for Dissociation (Adult): www.isst-d.org/resources/adult
-treatment-guidelines
Treatment Guidelines for Dissociation (Child/Adolescent): www.isst-d.org
/resources/child-adolescent-treatment-guidelines

Podcasts

10 Percent Happier
The Adult Chair
The Dope Black Therapist Podcast
The Heumann Perspective
Mindset Mentor

The Modern Therapist's Survival Guide
Psychologists Off the Clock
The Psychology Podcast
Small Things Often
Stuck Not Broken
System Speak
Therapist Uncensored
The Trauma Therapist Podcast

Apps

Calm
Insight Timer
Simply Plural

Books (Memoir)

A Fractured Mind: My Life with Multiple Personality Disorder by Robert Oxnam
Got Parts? An Insider's Guide to Managing Life Successfully with Dissociative Identity Disorder by A.T.W.
If Tears Were Prayers by Emma Sunshaw
The Magic Daughter: A Memoir of Living with Multiple Personality Disorder by Jane Phillips
Nobody Nowhere by Donna Williams
Recovery Is My Best Revenge: My Experience of Trauma, Abuse, and Dissociative Identity Disorder by Carolyn Spring
The Sum of My Parts: A Survivor's Story of Dissociative Identity Disorder by Olga Trujillo
Untamed by Glennon Doyle
When Rabbit Howls by (the Troops for) Truddi Chase

Books (Fiction or Expressive Arts)

Body Aware by Erica Hornthal
Carnival Lights by Chris Stark
Daily Medicine: 365 Days of Spiritual Meditations by Wayne William Snellgrove
My Mommy Has Multiple Parts by Joh Knyn
Nickels: A Tale of Dissociation by Christine Stark
Parts Work: An Illustrated Guide to Your Inner Life by Tom Holmes
Poetry, Prose, and Miscellaneous Musings by Kellie Kirksey
Process Not Perfection: Expressive Arts Solutions for Trauma Recovery by Jamie Marich
Starship Therapise: Using Therapeutic Fanfiction to Rewrite Your Life by Larisa Garski and Justine Mastin

The Story of the Oyster and the Butterfly and All the Parts of Me by Ana Gomez
A Wizard of Earthsea by Ursula LaGuin
Word Medicine: Affirmations and Poems to Inspire Our Journey by Kellie Kirksey

Books (Informational)

Amongst Ourselves: A Self-Help Guide to Living with Dissociative Identity Disorder by Tracy Alderman and Karen Marshall

Atlas of the Heart by Brené Brown

Becoming Yourself: Overcoming Mind Control and Ritual Abuse by Alison Miller

The Body Keeps the Score: Brain, Mind, and Body in the Healing of Trauma by Bessel van der Kolk

The Body Never Lies: The Lingering Effects of Hurtful Parenting by Alice Miller

Complex PTSD: From Surviving to Thriving by Pete Walker

The Complex PTSD Treatment Manual: An Integrative, Mind-Body Approach to Trauma Recovery by Arielle Schwartz

Coping with Trauma-Related Dissociation: Skills Training for Patients and Therapists by Suzette Boon, Kathy Steele, and Onno van der Hart

Dissociation and the Dissociative Disorders: DSM-V and Beyond by Paul Dell and John O'Neill (Eds.)

Dissociation, Mindfulness, and Creative Meditations: Trauma-Informed Practices to Facilitate Growth by Christine Forner

The Dissociative Identity Disorder Sourcebook by Deborah Bray Haddock

The Drama of the Gifted Child: The Search for the True Self by Alice Miller

Easy Ego State Interventions: Strategies for Working with Parts by Robin Shapiro

Every Memory Deserves Respect: EMDR, the Proven Trauma Therapy with the Power to Heal by Michael Baldwin and Deborah Korn

Feed Your Demons by Lama Tsultrim Allione

The Four-Fold Way: Walking the Paths of the Warrior, Teacher, Healer, and Visionary by Angeles Arrien

Getting Past Your Past: Take Control of Your Life with Self-Help Techniques from EMDR Therapy by Francine Shapiro

The Haunted Self: Structural Dissociation and the Treatment of Chronic Traumatization by Onno van der Hart, Ellert Nijenhuis, and Kathy Steele

Healing the Fragmented Selves of Trauma Survivors: Overcoming Internal Self-Alienation by Janina Fisher

Leaving the Fold: A Guide for Former Fundamentalists and Others Leaving Their Religion by Marlene Winell

Me, Not-Me, and We: A Lived Experience Workbook for Phased Recovery from Complex and Relational Trauma with Dissociative Identity Response by Emma Sunshaw

Multiple Personality Disorder from the Inside Out by Barry Cohen, Esther Giller, and Lynn W. (Eds.)

A Mythic Life by Jean Houston

No Bad Parts: Healing Trauma and Restoring Wholeness with the Internal Family Systems Model by Richard Schwartz

Perspectives of Dissociative Identity Response: Ethical, Historical, and Cultural Issues by Emily Christensen

The Rape of Eve: The True Story Behind the Three Faces of Eve by Colin Ross

Seeking Safety: A Treatment Manual for PTSD and Substance Abuse by Lisa Najavits

The Stranger in the Mirror: Dissociation—The Hidden Epidemic by Marlene Steinberg and Maxine Schnall

This Is Your Mind on Plants by Michael Pollan

Trauma and Dissociation-Informed Psychotherapy: Relational Healing and the Therapeutic Connection by Elizabeth Howell

Trauma and the 12 Steps: An Inclusive Guide to Enhancing Recovery by Jamie Marich

Trauma Made Simple by Jamie Marich

The Trauma Toolkit: Healing PTSD from the Inside Out by Susan Pease Banitt

Treating Complex Traumatic Stress Disorder in Adults: Scientific Foundations and Therapeutic Models by Christine Courtois and Julian Ford

Treatment of Complex Trauma: A Sequenced, Relationship-Based Approach by Christine Courtois and Julian Ford

Treatment of Dissociative Identity Disorder: Techniques and Strategies for Stabilization by Colin Ross

Unshame: Healing Trauma-Based Shame through Psychotherapy by Carolyn Spring

The Way of the Shaman by Michael Harner

What Happened to You? Conversations on Trauma, Resilience, and Healing by Oprah Winfrey and Bruce Perry

Wisdom, Attachment and Love in Trauma Therapy: Beyond Evidence-Based Practice by Susan Pease Banitt

Articles

"Addiction as Dissociation Model," by Adam O'Brien and Jamie Marich, *The Institute for Creative Mindfulness Redefine Therapy Blog,* October 2019. www.instituteforcreativemindfulness.com/icm-blog-redefine-therapy /addiction-as-dissociation-model-by-adam-obrien-dr-jamie-marich

"Flashback Management in the Treatment of Complex PTSD," by Pete Walker, *The East Bay Therapist,* September/October 2005. www.pete-walker.com /flashbackManagement.htm

"Harvey Weinstein's 'False Memory' Defense and Its Shocking Origin Story," by Anna Holtzman, *Medium,* February 2020. https://medium.com/fourth-wave /harvey-weinsteins-false-memory-defense-and-its-shocking-origin-story -2b0e4b98d526

"How *Moon Knight* Plays Into Hollywood's Obsession with Dissociative Identity Disorder," by Charles Pullam-Moore, *The Verge,* April 27, 2022. www.theverge .com/2022/4/27/23031165/moon-knight-dissociative-identity-disorder-marvel -disney-plus?fbclid=IwAR0d6AbrSbm1JQoN0EZ1e-wXznxWrebUoYyco15y5j SoM6oOeN8pOv4M-U8

"Multi-Layered," by Adrian Fletcher, *Psychiatric Services* (A Journal of the American Psychiatric Association), March 4, 2022. https://ps.psychiatryonline.org /doi/10.1176/appi.ps.202100706

"Psychologists Are Starting to Talk Publicly About Their Own Mental Illness— And Patients Can Benefit," by Andrew Devendorf and Sarah Victor, *The Conversation,* April 29, 2022. https://theconversation.com/psychologists -are-starting-to-talk-publicly-about-their-own-mental-illnesses-and -patients-can-benefit-177716?fbclid=IwAR12e495ygxmyyYABsKtjTfH9ZsxUto KiHETIUxs5lHnZ7r8zdq2QIDlU2o

"Separating Fact from Fiction: An Empirical Examination of Six Myths About Dissociative Identity Disorder," by Bethany Brand, Vedat Sar, Pam Stavropoulous, Christa Kruger, Marilyn Korzekwa, Alfonso Martinez-Taboas, and Warwick Middleton, *Harvard Review of Psychiatry,* 2016. https://journals .lww.com/hrpjournal/Fulltext/2016/07000/Separating_Fact_from_Fiction __An_Empirical.2.aspx

Notes

Introduction

1　Dictionary.com, s.v. "complex," accessed December 28, 2021, www.dictionary
.com/browse/complex; Dictionary.com, s.v. "complexity," accessed December 28,
2021, www.dictionary.com/browse/complexity.

2　Michael Crotty, *The Foundations of Social Research: Meaning and Perspective in
the Research Process* (London: Sage Publications, 1998), 80.

3　Grant McCracken, *The Long Interview: Qualitative Research Methods,* Volume 13
(Newbury Park, CA: Sage Publications, 1988).

Chapter 1

1　James Fadiman and Jordan Gruber, *Your Symphony of Selves: Discover and
Understand More of Who You Are* (Rochester, VT: Park Street Press, 2020), 375.

2　Bethany L. Brand et al., "Separating Fact from Fiction: An Empirical Examination of Six Myths About Dissociative Identity Disorder, *Harvard Review of
Psychiatry* 24, no. 4 (2016): 257–270.

3　*28 Days,* directed by Betty Thomas (2000; USA: Columbia Pictures), DVD.

4　Adam O'Brien and Jamie Marich, "Addiction as Dissociation Model," in
Jamie Marich and Stephen Dansiger, *Healing Addiction with EMDR Therapy:
A Trauma-Focused Guide* (New York: Springer Publishing Company, 2022), 122.

5　Jamie Marich (Interview), "Dissociation: Sharing from a Personal Place," *Go
With That* 24, no. 2 (2019), 5–6.

6　Dictionary.com, s.v. "dissociation," accessed December 1, 2021, www.dictionary
.com/browse/dissociation.

Chapter 2

1 Valerie Richardson, "African American Museum Removes 'Whiteness' Chart Over Claims of Backhanded Racism," *The Washington Times,* July 17, 2020, www.washingtontimes.com/news/2020/jul/17/smithsonian-african-american -museum-remove-whitene.

2 Sand Chang (@heydrsand), "How Do We Define Evidence," Instagram, June 22, 2021, www.instagram.com/p/CQbnz82LUdP.

3 Rene Descartes, *Meditations on First Philosophy,* trans. Michael Moriarty, Oxford World's Classics (London: Oxford University Press, 2008).

4 Christina Sarich, "The Mind vs. Brain Debate (What is Consciousness?)," *The Cuyamungue Institute,* accessed June 11, 2015, www.cuyamungueinstitute .com/articles-and-news/the-mind-vs-brain-debate-what-is-consciousness.

5 Jamie Marich, *Dancing Mindfulness: A Creative Path to Healing and Transformation* (Woodstock, VT: SkylightPaths Publishing, 2015), 67.

6 Foreword by Stephen Porges, in Deb Dana, *The Polyvagal Theory in Therapy* (New York, Norton Professional Books, 2020): xiii–xvii.

7 Deb Dana, *Polyvagal Exercises for Safety and Connection: 50 Client-Centered Practices* (New York: W.W. Norton & Company, 2020), 10–14.

8 O'Brien and Marich, "Addiction as Dissociation Model," 122.

9 Robert D. Ashford, Austin Brown, Jessica McDaniel, and Brenda Curtis, "Biased Labels: An Experimental Study of Language and Stigma among Individuals in Recovery and Health Professionals," *Substance Use and Misuse* 54, no. 4 (2019), 1376–1384.

10 Ellert Nijenhuis and Onno van der Hart, "Dissociation in Trauma: A New Definition and Comparison with Previous Formulations," *Journal of Trauma and Dissociation* 12, no. 4 (2011), 418.

11 Nijenhuis and van der Hart, "Dissociation in Trauma."

12 Nijenhuis and van der Hart, "Dissociation in Trauma."

13 Michaela Mergler et al., "Relationship between a Dissociative Subtype of PTSD and Clinical Characteristics in Patients with Substance Use Disorders," *Journal of Psychoactive Drugs* 49, no. 3 (2017), 225–232.

14 Bessel van der Kolk, "The Compulsion to Repeat the Trauma: Re-enactment, Revictimization, and Masochism," *Psychiatric Clinics of North America* 12 (1989), 389–411; Ulrich Lanius, "Dissociation and Endogenous Opioids: A Foundational Role," in *Neurobiology and Treatment of Traumatic Dissociation: Toward an Embodied Self,* ed. Ulrich Lanius, Sandra Paulsen, and Frank Corrigan (New York: Springer Publishing Company, 2014), 81–104.

15 *Lanius,* "Dissociation and Endogenous Opioids."

16 Paul F. Dell and John A. O'Neil, "The Long Struggle to Diagnose Multiple Personality Disorder (MPD): Partial MPD," in *Dissociation and the Dissociative*

Disorders: DSM-V and Beyond, ed. Paul F. Dell and John A. O'Neil (New York: Routledge, 2015), 383–402.

17 American Psychiatric Association, *Diagnostic and Statistical Manual of Mental Disorders* (DSM-5), 5th ed. (Arlington, VA: American Psychiatric Association, 2013), https://doi.org/10.1176/appi.books.9780890425596.

18 Christine Courtois and Julian Ford, *Treating Complex Traumatic Stress Disorders: An Evidence-Based Guide,* 2nd ed. (New York: Guilford Press, 2020), 1.

19 Judy Singer, *Neurodiversity: The Birth of an Idea,* eBook, 2017, www.neuroredux.blogspot.com.

20 In her 2022 article, Emily Christensen also makes this point and cites some of the emerging research in this area: Emily Christensen, "The Online Community: DID and Plurality," *European Journal of Trauma and Dissociation* 6, no. 2, (2022), https://doi.org/10.1016/j.ejtd.2021.100257.

21 Kathy Steele, Suzette Boon, and Onno van der Hart, *Treating Trauma-Related Dissociation: A Practical, Integrative Approach* (New York: W.W. Norton, 2017), 122.

Chapter 3

1 Christine Forner, "What Mindfulness Can Learn from Dissociation and What Dissociation Can Learn from Mindfulness," *Journal of Trauma and Dissociation* 20, no. 1 (2019), 1–15.

2 Martha Postlewaite, "Grounding: Coming into the Here and Now by Using Our Bodily Sensations," in *101 Interventions in Group Therapy,* ed. Scott Simon Fehr, 2nd ed. (New York: Routledge, 2016), 78–80.

3 Jon Kabat-Zinn, *Mindfulness for Beginners: Reclaiming the Present Moment—and Your Life* (Boulder, CO: Sounds True Books, 2012), 94.

4 Eliza Griswold, "Yoga Considers the Role of the Guru in the Age of #MeToo," *The New Yorker,* July 23, 2019, www.newyorker.com/news/news-desk/yoga-reconsiders-the-role-of-the-guru-in-the-age-of-metoo; Gemma Bath, "Kidnapping, Sexual Abuse, and Lies: The Dark History of Yoga's Introduction to the West," *MamaMia,* June 24, 2020, www.mamamia.com.au/yoga-scandals; Katherine Rosman, "Yoga is Finally Facing Consent and Unwanted Touch," *The New York Times,* November 15, 2019, www.nytimes.com/2019/11/08/style/yoga-touch-consent-harassment.html.

5 Tsultrim Allione, *Feed Your Demons* (New York: Little, Brown, 2008).

6 John A. O'Brien, "The Healing of Nations," *Psychological Perspectives* 60, no. 2 (2017), 207–214.

7 Claire Frederick and Shirley McNeal, *Inner Strengths: Contemporary Psychotherapy and Hypnosis for Ego Strengthening* (New York: Routledge, 2014), 77.

8 George Fraser, "The Dissociative Table Technique: A Strategy for Working with Ego States in Dissociative Disorders and Ego State Therapy,"

Dissociation 4, no. 4 (1991), 205–213; George Fraser, "Fraser's 'Dissociative Table Technique' Revisited, Revised: A Strategy for Working with Ego States in Dissociative Disorders and Ego State Therapy," *Journal of Trauma and Dissociation* 4, no. 4 (2003), 5–28.

9 Onno van der Hart, Ellert Nijenhuis, and Kathy Steele, *The Haunted Self: Structural Dissociation and the Treatment of Chronic Traumatization* (New York: W.W. Norton & Company, 2006).

10 Colin Ross, *Structural Dissociation: A Proposed Modification of the Theory* (Richardson, TX: Manitou Communications, 2013).

11 Richard Schwartz and Martha Sweezy, *Internal Family Systems Therapy,* 2nd ed. (New York: Guilford Press, 2019).

12 Frank Anderson, *Transcending Trauma: Healing Complex PTSD with Internal Family Systems* (Eau Claire, WI: PESI Publishing, 2021), 21.

Chapter 5

1 Jamie Marich, "A Personal (and Professional) Take on Dissociative Disorders," *The Mighty,* December 4, 2018, https://themighty.com/2018/12/dissociative -disorders-professional-personal-perspective.

2 Daniel Siegel, *The Developing Mind: How Relationships and the Brain Interact to Shape Who We Are* (New York: Guilford Press, 1999).

3 Katarina Lundgren, "The Wheel of Tolerance," *Live the Change,* December 7, 2019, https://livethechange.se/index.php/blog/the-wheel-of-tolerance.

4 Kimberlé Crenshaw, "Decriminalizing the Intersection of Race and Sex: A Black Feminist Critique of Antidiscrimination Doctrine, Feminist Theory, and Racist Politics," *University of Chicago Legal Forum* no. 1, article 8 (1989), https://chicagounbound.uchicago.edu/cgi/viewcontent.cgi?article =1052&context=uclf.

5 Jane Coaston, "The Intersectionality Wars," *Vox,* May 28, 2019, www.vox.com /the-highlight/2019/5/20/18542843/intersectionality-conservatism-law-race -gender-discrimination.

Chapter 6

1 Francine Shapiro, *Eye Movement Desensitization and Reprocessing (EMDR): Basic Principles, Protocols, and Procedures,* 3rd ed. (New York: Guilford Press, 2018).

2 Onno van der Hart, Paul Brown, and Bessel van der Kolk, "Pierre Janet's Treatment of Post-Traumatic Stress," *Journal of Traumatic Stress* 2, no. 4 (1989), 1–11.

3 World Health Organization, *Assessment and Management of Conditions Specifically Related to Stress mhGAP Intervention Guide Module* (Geneva, Switzerland: World Health Organization, 2013), http://apps.who.int/iris/bitstream/10665 /85623/1/9789241505932_eng.pdf?ua=1.

4 Esther da Waal, "The Celtic Way of Prayer," *Spirituality and Practice: Resources for Spiritual Journeys,* n.d., www.spiritualityandpractice.com/quotes/quotations/view/10576/spiritual-quotation.

5 *The Wisdom of Trauma,* directed by Zaya Benazzo and Mauricio Benazzo (2021; USA: Science and Nonduality), feature film.

6 Lisa Jerome, et al., "Long-Term Follow-Up Outcomes of MDMA-Assisted Psychotherapy for Treatment of PTSD: A Longitudinal Pooled Analysis of Six Phase 2 Trials," *Psychopharmacology* 237, no. 8 (2020), 2485–2497; Kai Kupferschmidt, "All Clear for the Decisive Trial of Ecstasy in PTSD Patients," *Science,* August 26, 2017, www.science.org/content/article/all-clear-decisive-trial-ecstasy-ptsd-patients.

7 Michael Pollan, *This Is Your Mind on Plants* (New York: Penguin Press, 2021), 11.

Chapter 7

1 Brand et al., "Separating Fact from Fiction," 257–270.

2 Onno van der Hart and Andrew Moskowitz, "Multiple States of Consciousness, Complexes, Personalities, or Parts of the Personality? An Historical Perspective and Contemporary Proposal on Trauma-Related Dissociation," *Rivista Sperimentale di Freniatria* 1 (2018), 51–71.

3 Anna Holtzman, "Harvey Weinstein's 'False Memory' Defense and Its Shocking Origin Story: How Powerful Sex Offenders Manipulated the Field of Psychology," *Fourth Wave,* February 13, 2020, https://medium.com/fourth-wave/harvey-weinsteins-false-memory-defense-and-its-shocking-origin-story-2b0e4b98d526.

4 Jamie Marich, "Dear Ryan Murphy: Your Portrayal of This Mental Disorder in *Ratched* is Damaging," *The Mighty,* October 16, 2020, https://themighty.com/2020/10/ratched-dissociative-identity-disorder-charlotte-wrong.

5 *Adam B. Vary,* "How 'Moon Knight' Sends Marvel Studios Into the Unknown: 'We're Creating a Whole New Thing,'" *Variety,* archived *from the original March 31, 2022, accessed* March 31, 2022.

6 Jessica Lucas, "Inside TikTok's Booming Dissociative Identity Disorder Community," *Input,* July 6, 2021, www.inputmag.com/culture/dissociative-identity-disorder-did-tiktok-influencers-multiple-personalities.

7 Emily Christensen, "The Online Community: DID and Plurality," *European Journal of Trauma & Dissociation* 6, no. 2, (2022), https://doi.org/10.1016/j.ejtd.2021.100257.

8 Mike Hilleary, "Counting Crows' Adam Duritz on Nostalgia, Dissociative Disorder and His Band's New EP," *InsideHook,* May 21, 2021, www.insidehook.com/article/music/counting-crows-adam-duritz-interview

9 Anderson, *Transcending Trauma,* 21.

Conclusion

1 A. Mark Williams and Tim Wigmore, "Under Pressure: Why Athletes Choke," *The Guardian,* November 5, 2020, www.theguardian.com/sport/2020/nov/05 /under-pressure-why-athletes-choke.

Appendix A for Clinicians and Therapists

1 Brand et al., "Separating Fact from Fiction."
2 Anaïs Nin and Paul Herron, *The Quotable Anaïs Nin* (San Antonio, TX: Blue Sky Press), 92.

Index

About the Author

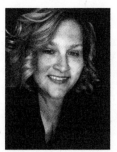

Dr. Jamie+ Marich (she/they) describes themselves as a facilitator of transformative experiences. A clinical trauma specialist, expressive artist, writer, yogini, performer, short filmmaker, reiki master, TEDx speaker, and recovery advocate, she unites all of these elements in her mission to inspire healing in others. Jamie is a woman in long-term recovery from an addictive disorder and is living loudly and proudly as a woman with a dissociative disorder with the goal of smashing stigma about dissociation in the mental health field and in society at large.

Jamie began her career as a humanitarian aid worker in Bosnia-Herzegovina from 2000–2003, primarily teaching English and music. She travels internationally teaching on topics related to trauma, EMDR Therapy, expressive arts, mindfulness, and yoga, while maintaining a private practice and online education operations in her home base of northeast Ohio. Jamie is the founder of The Institute for Creative Mindfulness and the developer of the Dancing Mindfulness approach to expressive arts therapy. She is the author of *EMDR Made Simple: 4 Approaches for Using EMDR with Every Client* (2011); *Trauma and the Twelve Steps: A Complete Guide to Enhancing Recovery* (2012); *Creative Mindfulness* (2013); *Trauma Made Simple: Competencies in Assessment, Treatment, and Working with Survivors* (2014); *Dancing Mindfulness: A Creative Path to Healing and Transformation* (2015); and *Process Not Perfection: Expressive Arts Solutions for Trauma Recovery* (2019). Jamie coauthored *EMDR Therapy & Mindfulness for Trauma-Focused Care* along with colleague Dr. Stephen Dansiger in 2018, and their second book with Springer Publishing, *Healing Addiction with EMDR Therapy: A Trauma-Focused Guide,* was published in 2021. North Atlantic Books published a revised and expanded edition of *Trauma and the 12 Steps* in summer

2020, and also published *The Healing Power of Jiu-Jitsu: A Guide to Transforming Trauma and Facilitating Recovery* (with Anna Pirkl). The *New York Times* featured Jamie's writing and work on *Dancing Mindfulness* in 2017 and 2020. NALGAP: The Association of Lesbian, Gay, Bisexual, Transgender Addiction Professionals and Their Allies awarded Jamie with their esteemed President's Award in 2015 for her work as an LGBT advocate. The EMDR International Association (EMDRIA) granted Jamie the 2019 Advocacy in EMDR Award for her using her public platform in the media and in the addiction field to advance awareness about EMDR Therapy and to reduce stigma around mental health.

About North Atlantic Books

North Atlantic Books (NAB) is an independent, nonprofit publisher committed to a bold exploration of the relationships between mind, body, spirit, and nature. Founded in 1974, NAB aims to nurture a holistic view of the arts, sciences, humanities, and healing. To make a donation or to learn more about our books, authors, events, and newsletter, please visit www.northatlanticbooks.com.